REF
RA
790.6
•M447 Mental health
services in
transition

DATE			
	DISCARD		

MENTAL HEALTH SERVICES
IN TRANSITION

MENTAL HEALTH SERVICES IN TRANSITION

A Policy Sourcebook

Edited by
Theodore R. Vallance
The Pennsylvania State University
University Park, PA

Ru M. Sabre
University of Tennessee
Chattanooga, TN

HUMAN SCIENCES PRESS, INC.
72 Fifth Avenue   3 Henrietta Street
NEW YORK, NY 10011 ● LONDON, WC2E 8LU

This publication is made possible through the support of a grant from the National Institute of Mental Health No. 5 T 21 MH 13484.

Library of Congress Cataloging in Publication Data

Mental health services in transition.

  Based on presentations made at a colloquium in the graduate program in community systems planning and development, Pennsylvania State University.
  1. Community mental health services—Government policy—United States—Congresses.
I. Vallance, Theodore R. II. Sabre, Ru M. [DNLM: 1. Community mental health services—
Trends—Congresses.   WM M5532 1973-74]
RA790.6.M447   362.2'0973   81-6805
ISBN 0-87705-700-1   AACR2

CONTRIBUTORS

Theodore R. Vallance has been Professor of Human Development at Penn State's College of Human Development since 1967, and Associate Dean for Research and Graduate Study until 1979. Dr. Vallance holds joint appointment in the Departments of Community Development and of Man-Environment Relations and is on the faculty of the graduate program in Community Systems Planning and Development. Prior to going to Penn State he was Chief of the Office of Planning at the National Institute of Mental Health.

Ru M. Sabre is Associate Professor of Human Services in the University of Tennessee at Chattanooga. His doctorate is in Community Systems Planning and Development from Penn State. Prior to resuming graduate study at Penn State Dr. Sabre taught philosophy at Guilford College.

Bruce L. Baker, Professor of Psychology, University of California at Los Angeles.

William B. Beach, Jr., Director, Brattleboro Retreat, Professor of Psychology and Chief, Division of Child Psychiatry, Dartmouth Medical School, formerly Commissioner of Mental Health, Commonwealth of Pennsylvania.

Anthony Broskowski, Executive Director, Northside Community Mental Health Center, Inc., Tampa, Florida.

W. Louis Coppersmith, Senator, Pennsylvania Legislature, Chairman, Committee on Health and Welfare.

Terry Dellmuth, Former Special Assistant to the Governer for Human Services, Commonwealth of Pennsylvania.

Gunnar Dybwad, Professor Emeritus of Human Development, Brandeis University.

Frederick R. Eisele, Associate Professor of Social Policy, Graduate Program in Community Systems Planning and Development, The Pennsylvania State University.

Ira Goldenberg, Dean, Human Services Department, New Hampshire College.

Bernard Guerney, Jr., Professor of Human Development, The Pennsylvania State University.

Marcia Guttentag, Deceased. Formerly lecturer on Education, Harvard University.

Leonard Hassol, Professor of Psychology, Wheaton College.

James G. Kelley, Professor of Psychology, The School of Community Services and Public Affairs, The University of Oregon.

Lewis B. Klebanoff, Deputy Assistant Commissioner for Mental Retardation, Commonwealth of Massachusets.

Adeline Levine, Associate Professor of Sociology, State University of New York at Buffalo.

Murray Levine, Professor of Psychology, State University of New York at Buffalo.

Robert Reiff, Psychologist, President of Sparc Institute, Austin, Texas.

Lucille Robuck, former chairman, Parole Board, Commonwealth of Kentucky; currently Associate Professor of Law Enforcement, Eastern Kentucky University.

Grove A. Spearly, Sr., Commissioner of Centre County, Pennsylvania.

Charles Windle, Program Evaluation Specialist, National Institute of Mental Health.

CONTENTS

7

PREFACE

It is easy to overlook the fact that significant social movements are powered by the enthusiasm and commitment of people in what becomes known in later years as "the field" and finally as a public policy area. This book is a source for understanding the community mental health movement and its relations with other human services. More importantly, it conveys a sense of the personalities within the significant institutional and societal roles that make the community mental health movement what it is and is not.

The present volume grew out of a colloquium in the graduate program in Community Systems Planning and Development at The Pennsylvania State University. The series was a National Institute of Mental Health supported effort which addressed the topic of incorporating mental health concepts in social policy planning. We saw an opportunity to perform two important services by editing and organizing the speakers' presentations. The spoken presentations conveyed a considerable amount of practical wisdom, a view of the working contexts and conflicts in which the community mental health movement has grown, and a frankness that we feel we have preserved in the translation from the spoken to the written word. We also saw the talks as providing a breadth and depth of vision into the wide range of issues which form the mental health program effort.

A great amount of information is presented in an organized manner on many aspects of mental health services. The articles range over such issue areas as the history and development of the community mental health movement, how mental health concerns fare in state legislatures, in the county commissioners' and the governor's offices, and the efforts to evaluate and change the value set of those involved in the mental health and human service area. We are pleased that whatever the topic, in each case human concern for human problems is the guiding principle of the presentations.

This book is clearly the result of the interest and effort of many people. The names of several of them do not appear in the table of contents. Drs. Ralph Simon, Samuel Silverstein, and Beatrice Shriver of the National Institute of Mental Health helped to shape some of the concepts of the grant of funds that underwrote the basic expenses of the book and provided major support for the educational program in which the book developed. Dr. Silverstein especially provided help and encouragement in the publication stages of the work. Essential editorial work of rendering roughly edited transcriptions of the presentations into readable prose was accomplished by Marque Bagshaw. The difficult work of transcribing the frequently disjointed oral presentations was the responsibility of Sherry Sharum, who also did much of the final typing. Special thanks are due to Martha Stouffer, who completed the manuscript and efficiently took care of the numberless details in getting the project finally ready for publication.

HISTORICAL BACKDROP: SOME HUMAN PROBLEMS AND WAYS OF DEALING WITH THEM

One of the strangest qualities of modern society is that decisions which affect the lives of millions of people are made by people who are essentially "invisible" and immune to the broad consequences of these decisions. Once an official becomes part of some subcommittee this *individual* is no longer making the decisions. Responsibility is dissolved in the dynamics of group interaction and compromise. Further, the administration of any business or social program can always scapegoat some administrator but the public knows that justice has not been done.

A major goal of this book is to bring attention to the various administrators, bureaucrats, and politicians as *people* involved and concerned with those affected by their decisions. We are trying to present voices of concern within the vast human service bureaucracies.

It is our conviction that in order to cope with and to alter bureaucratic momentum, it is necessary to understand the decision makers as people under the stress of reconciling personal commitment, procedural complexity, and environmental uncertainty. It is also necessary to understand the historical development of organized efforts to deal with social problems, and what the current trends are. Some social critics would call this a whitewash, asserting that we are just trying to persuade or dupe the public into the view that no better job could be done; that we are just saying here, look at these people, could you do a better job? Our answer is that nothing can be done without adequate knowledge, and that a critical dimension of that knowledge is an understanding of the personal dimension of decision making and evaluation by people who have made a life's work out of trying to implement an organized assault on social problems.

Historians of human services have noted that the disadvantaged face a two-way road to Hell paved with good intentions. In good times, the people who receive subsidized human services are seen as failing because of a lack of initiative or some personal quality that makes the individual person responsible for his or her failure. Programs are launched and funded that stress individual rehabilitation. Just as these programs are stabilizing and becoming part of the institutional structure, the national economy takes a turn for the worse and the perception of the disadvantaged population changes. Now they are seen as victims of their environment, and the idea emerges that what is needed is an improved environment for the individuals—they need a wider range of choices. The "solution" of the prosperous times becomes the problem of the belt tightening phase of the economy. For funds are now committed to the opposite point of view and much time is consumed in bureaucratic infighting to change the policy structure.

Perhaps nowhere is this historical dilemma more evident than in the mental hospital as the catch-all solution to a particular class of the disadvantaged—those who have been mentally ill. The state legislature is in charge of its mental hospitals. They came into being in the prosperous times at the end of the nineteenth century as part of a reform movement aimed at the barbaric treatment of these people. What to do with people who simply cannot live in society was the problem to which mental hospitals were the solution. In an environment where individual initiative was seen as the necessary condition for living and succeeding in society, what is to be done with people who are incapable of engaging in the competitive struggle? The inheritance of contemporary state legislatures is the need to balance off individual rights and institutional needs. Involuntary commitment is the epitome of that problem.

State legislators are caught between the unions and professional service providers' demands for clients and the moral imperative to allow the individual to stay in a social setting which just might catch and draw him back to normality. The legislation that allows for involuntary commitment is shaped by these potentially contrary forces. How does one legislate in such a way as to constrain those who need institutionalization and keep free those who do not? It is easy to overlook the fact that the dilemma exists because there exist such institutions as mental hospitals which constrain and shape people for different reasons.

Taken from a broader perspective, there exists a significant professional, political, and union pressure to preserve the mental hospital. William Beach summarizes the experience of two states in coping with these pressures. Parallel social pressures for similar reasons are operative in correctional facilities. Lucille Robuck emphasizes the need to help the paroled or discharged convict when he returns to the community. The types of counseling needed stress community-based services and the latter display the irrelevance of the state hospital to the state correctional facility. In a world where institutions are launching strategic offenses to preserve particular interests, the voice of the prophet is not unwelcome. Gunnar Dybwad in unequivocal terms spells out the horrors of institutional life. Stressing the values of individual dignity and the worth of every individual, his call to conscience cannot be ignored by any contending faction. Indeed, the rhetoric of the competing groups is often cast in the form of what is "best" for the individual. There is no doubt, though, that the right to education and to treatment for retardates would not exist without his outside advocacy.

Chapter 1

MENTAL HEALTH AND SOCIAL STRUCTURE: AN OVERVIEW AND INTRODUCTION TO THE CURRENT SCENE

Theodore R. Vallance
Ru M. Sabre

Society's stepchild could be blind, crippled, insane, poor, an orphan, an alcoholic, drug-dependent, starving, unemployed, or have any other characteristic which gives the person the appearance of deviating from the norm. Social Darwinists call them "rejects" or "culls"; social humanitarians call them disadvantaged human beings who need help. By whatever name, social welfare forms a field whose function is to administer to the needs of these people and will continue to play a part in our complex urbanized society. This book attempts to evoke a picture of the current status of the helping services and forecast in a policy relevant way its future.

A brief look at the history of the helping services informs us about the origins of present attitudes which linger on and continue to shape the nature of services. There is historical truth to the notion that in the West, organized assistance to those in need can be divided into three historically defined epochs: (1) from Charlemagne's Empire in 800 AD to the founding of nation states and the great religious wars of the 1500s; (2) from the Elizabethan Poor Laws of 1601 to the Great Depression of the 1930s; and (3) from the Social Security Act of 1935 to the present, a period of 45 years. These epochs reflect the great political and economic transitions in the West: the shift from the medieval period to the industrialized nation state, the development of the nation state up to World War II, and the attendant realignment of world powers and interacting ideologies that form the essence of the modern world.

In the feudal period, the Church and the feudal lord took total responsibility for the needy. The monastery was in reality a multiservice center caring for the needs of both body and soul. The breakdown of the medieval synthesis with the shift of economic and political power going to the nation state created enormous problems in the developing urban areas. The Elizabethan Poor Laws of 1601 provided that (1) local authorities be given the power to tax for the relief of the poor; (2) the local authorities could set up overseers of the poor to administer to the poor; (3) the overseers could provide assistance to the needy in their homes or, if homeless, could provide work houses where the strong might work; (4) the employable must work; (5) the overseer could take indigents back to their place of birth, that place being the locus of responsibility for that person in need; (6) parents were expected to care for their children, and children for their parents; and (7) children at the age of four might be indentured to learn a trade.

These poor laws attempted to deal with abuses within the existing system, but they went virtually unchanged for the next 300 years. English common law became the law of the American colonies. In this period of time, the West experienced the forces of industrialization, urbanization, and colonization. Emigration became a major means of dealing with many of the needy, with those who did not fit into the functioning aspects of society, for whatever reason. This second epoch culminated in the political, economic, and social upheaval of the 1930s.

One response of the United States to the Great Depression was the Social Security Act of 1935. The formation and growth of the Department of Health, Education and Welfare since the end of World War II bears witness to the magnitude of the governmental response of this country to the disadvantaged.

The most recent chapters in the development of the 1935 act are the Health Systems Agency legislation and the new Title XX of the Social Security Act. The Health Systems Agency legislation attempts to create effective regional planning bodies responsible for providing maximum health service delivery while holding down costs. The new Title XX provided for the first time in our history a flat sum of money (in 1975–1976 it was $2.5 billion) specifically for social services associated with the local boards of public assistance.

These and other current pieces of legislation are designed to meet the problems brought about by the competition between and the confusion within local service delivery agencies. Competition and confusion exist today primarily because social welfare programs came into being within federal bureaucracies which themselves started programs independently of other departments' efforts. These various categorical programs converge on the local level through a state bureaucracy which in the past has acted as a politically structured conduit of funds for local agencies. Research into means of dealing with program fragmentation and costly duplication can be seen as part of the recent attempt to restructure the conduit by using program coordination or integration as goals.

The variety of programs intersecting on the local (county, borough, city) level is illustrative of service coordination problems at the local delivery level: family planning, legal aid, youth services, aging programs, child development councils, child welfare, community action, meals on wheels, home health services, public health, interfaces with the board of assistance, probation and parole, juvenile courts, sheltered workshops of all types, local planning councils, county jails, nursing homes, vocational schools, intermediate units, rehabilitation centers, urban renewal, group homes, halfway houses, hotline services, citizen advocacy groups, clergy consultation services, public hearings, PTA, ministerial associations, civil defense, consumer services, domestic relations, drug and alcohol abuse programs, veterans affairs, United Way, tuberculosis and respiratory programs, combined mental health and mental retardation (MH/ MR) programs and many others.

Local agencies have to deal with as many sets of eligibility criteria as there are programs, which has led to the call for coordination and integration of services. Recent experiences in program coordination have revealed coordination to be a concept that ill-fits the reality of human service delivery problems on the local level. The costs associated with an administrative umbrella over human service agencies are large, and the fundamental question has been raised of what benefits will be derived from the creation of yet another bureaucracy? Program coordination might also have a negative impact on the esprit de corps of voluntary organizations. These and other questions reveal that human services as a response to social ills can and ought to be seen and analyzed from an historical and developmental perspective, a perspective which this book develops. We are dealing with one broad subset of programs, that is, the mental health and mental retardation programs, but these programs are a focus within the general area of the helping services.

In its inception in 1963, the Community Mental Health Centers Act is one more categorical program designed to address specific problems within the field of mental health service delivery, but which soon took on the community action flavor of the Great Society programs of the 1960s. The Act was to help relocate people who had been institutionalized to other settings and to prevent the institutionalization of those who were undergoing mental illnesses; in effect, to provide for those mentally ill individuals on the local level, people who might otherwise be exiled to a state mental hospital. The community action phase of mental health developed when the concept of prevention was seen as intimately tied to the deliberate change of local social arrangements.

The notion of locating rehabilitation at the community level has an historical evolution originating in the nineteenth century dungeons of Europe and America. In the early twentieth century, mental hospitals became feudal baronies with valuable land holdings, prize dairy herds, and self-sustaining agricultural activity. These conditions soon degenerated to warehousing and by the 1950s scandalous conditions and exorbitant costs resulted in a series of inquiries. Commission studies resulted in the community mental health movement as a strategy for returning closer to their home some of the exiled, treating various types of psychological breakdown immediately without prolonged isolation from society, and devising strategies for organizational and community intervention which would foster alterations of the social structure that would promote mental health.

The dual tasks of reintegration and prevention, however, involve the mental health center in coordinated efforts with other human services. The political realities of such coordination exist as different sets of problems on the local, state, and federal levels. When the state divides the funds which sustain agencies for the aging, child welfare, mental health, mental retardation, probation, and parole services, etc., tremendous pressures are brought to bear on county commissioners and on state officials. How can coordination and cooperation stand against the hard realities of budgetary demands made by agency executives who are each fighting for what each considers to be essential services?

In principle, the bargaining position of any human service agency will be strengthened if that agency can demonstrate that it is working efficiently and effectively. This is the task of good evaluation, a task which amounts to a quantitative accountability tied to some criteria indicative of the degree to which an agency is meeting its goals. Evaluation is a strategy that enables the federal bureaucracy to measure the performance of the state and local levels, and the state to measure the effectiveness and efficiency of local agencies, and to help local elected officials justify to their constituencies the ways in which they have used public resources entrusted to their care. Evaluation is also a means, in principle, by which an efficient and effective agency can form a basis for continued funding.

We suspect that it is quite unlikely that a wholly nonpolitical basis will be developed for dollar allocations, or even for evaluation. We might conclude by noting that good evaluation can *supplement* the crass aspects of political decision making and even strike a blow for rationality over the long haul. We could also, in so doing, caution against too high hopes for evaluation.

In effect, good evaluation can supplement the other criteria which politicians, bureaucrats, and agency executives seem to find necessary in policy making. The ideal logic of evaluation implies an instrument which tells the administrator how much money is being spent, but it is another thing to have an evaluation process which also helps the team delivering services do a better job. Nevertheless, in response to the call for accountability, evaluation efforts will play an important part in the structuring of human services planning and implementation.

The future of mental health services is intimately tied to that of the other helping services. With mental health services acting as the foreground of the general gestalt of human services, we hope to provide a basis for the projection of mental health concerns into human service planning. The historical-developmental pattern of this volume provides such a basis.

The section headings form the structure of this pattern. In Section I, a brief history of the helping services is provided by people who are both scholars and practitioners in the helping services. Two historians of social services provide a fascinating narrative depicting the American experience in general, while a lawyer and master tactician of the courts provides a particular focus in the Pennsylvania suit for the educational rights of the mentally retarded. From this historical milieu, the concept of community mental health services developed into an historical reality. In Section II this development is recounted by people who started to move the concept into reality. We provide here first hand accounts of the landmark conference at Swampscott. Here, the concept of community mental health was given clearer definition, of the mental health movement's forced maturation under the impulse of social action in the 1960s, and a timely far reaching critique of the movement.

Section III details the operational and political environment in which community mental health grew up. Here people of wide experience and deep concern provide insight, wisdom, and, most valuable of all, hope. The political realities of rationally and compassionately administering human services on the county, municipal, state, and federal level are explained by people who have years of experience in dealing with those problems.

In Section IV, researchers presently involved in the delivery and evaluation of mental health services discuss the consultation process, the diffusion of developmental skills, a self-help program for the parents of a retarded child, the dilemmas of evaluation, and the controversy over techniques for evaluating mental health services.

While it is true that social *theorists* have moved beyond social Darwinism and have realized the injustice of "blaming the victim," social *practice* seems to be slower in changing. As a step in that direction, we attempt to call attention to the nature of the value transition. A social contract point of view in fact provides an ethical basis for helping individuals, a basis which cannot be provided by the currently assumed utilitarian ethos. In the latter part of this section, we make observations about the value implications of a social contract ethic for human service operations which entail a stronger emphasis on individual and community developmental strategies.

Murray and Adeline Levine, historians of the human services, summarize the trends and movements leading to the present set of human services and offer some speculation about the future. Periods of renewed concern for people in which social reform movements offset the helping services, they say, seem to emphasize the spark of the divine in man with blame for human adversity going to the environment "out there." In periods of conservation, the blame seems to fall on the failing humans themselves and programs tend to become mainly rehabilitation. They believe that the reforms of the 1960s were aborted by the Vietnam war and speculate that reform movements will be seen again in five or ten years if meeting energy problems does not excessively consume economic resources.

Chapter 2

LONG-TERM TRENDS—ORIGINS OF MAJOR FORMS AND ASSOCIATED ISSUES*

Murray Levine
Adeline Levine

Human services are imbedded in the historical and social context of their time, and they develop and change in relation to that context. While we pride ourselves on our objectivity and the empirical base of our work, the set of variables we have included in our theories of providing help is really too narrow to deal with either the delivery of services or our conceptions of the nature of the mental health problem. The development of a community-based child guidance clinic will provide a case study to illustrate the issues.

Prehistory

The child guidance clinic developed in its modern form in the mid-1920s, but in order to understand the child guidance clinics of the 1920s, one needs to understand the previous 50- or 60-year period.

---

*This paper was based on the book *A Social History of Helping Services* (New York, Appleton- Century Crofts, 1970) by Adeline and Murray Levine. A different version of this lecture was previously published under the title "The More Things Change . . . A Case History of Child Guidance Clinics" in the *Journal of Social Issues* 1970, *26*, 3 (summer), 19–34.

Immediately after the Civil War, a period of rapid industrial expansion accompanied by massive immigration and continuing urbanization characterized the United States. After 1890, the frontier closed, and the new immigrants were packed into cities.

Overcrowded slums, poverty, poor working conditions, broken families, loss of family, and face-to-face community ties created a breeding ground for social problems. In that period, delinquency climbed, prostitution festered, welfare problems were intense, and school problems were widespread. Urban recreation facilities were largely absent. The American urban Protestant churches were losing influence because their constituencies were moving out to the suburbs, and the new immigrants coming in were all Catholics and Jews.

The political and economic systems were also under drastic pressure to change. After the 1890s, the corrupt municipal political machines came under attack, and efforts were made to obtain real reforms in housing, sanitation, and food inspection; in health, recreational, and educational facilities; and in the very inadequate system of individual, private philanthropy under which much of welfare was conducted. Most of the major professional facilities which focused upon child development and child welfare originated in this period between 1890 and 1912.

Ideology and Human Services

In the period of economic growth immediately following the Civil War, the dominant social ideology that justified reality was conservative Social Darwinism. This ideology stated that the social order had evolved because it was the best of all possible forms. Anybody who rose to the top was there because it was an evolutionary necessity, and anybody who was in unfortunate circumstances was innately inferior. Given that philosophy, it was folly to do anything to help the unfortunate because that encouraged the survival of weak forms of life threatening the very viability of society itself.

With this ideology the poor, the insane, or the criminal were viewed as unalterably less fit. Scientific charity was developed to distinguish the few worthy poor, the few people who were in need not of their own making, from the mass of the unworthy poor. It is little wonder that the helping agencies of that period were sometimes more punitive than helpful.

In the late 1880s and following, as the human problems became more disturbing to the social order, a different social philosophy became dominant. This viewpoint held that all people were innately good, that all had a potential for development, that if people had troubles it was the consequences of conditions around them. One helped people by changing the conditions of life. So the predominant helping forms of this period then consisted of providing new opportunities for people.

Predecessors to the Modern Clinic

The 20-year period preceding World War I saw the development of the two immediate predecessors of the child guidance clinics. Both were responsive to urban problems, and both developed as attempts to modify existing social institutions. The two are Lightner Witmer's Psychological Clinic, which was established in the Department of Psychology of the University of Pennsylvania in 1896, and William Healy's clinic, which was established as part of the first juvenile court in Chicago in 1909.

Witmer's theoretical emphasis was not so much on psychopathology as upon devising methods to permit the fullest emotional and intellectual development of those who were not being served educationally. In Witmer's view, it was the school and the educational facilities that needed to develop new methods to deal with the problems presented by people having different educational needs.

The juvenile courts were established on the premise that the prevalent treatment of juveniles as criminals contributed to their later development as adult criminals. The juvenile court was designed to change the legal treatment of children from one of punishment for crime to one in which the delinquent child would be dealt with by the state "as a wise parent would deal with a wayward child." The very function of a criminal court was changed in the development of the juvenile court. The juvenile court relied very heavily on a system of probation, the idea of giving the individual another chance. And probation workers, at least the early ones, saw it as their duty to deal with the social conditions that caused or fostered delinquency.

Healy's Clinic, established in 1909, was a result of citizens and probation officers working together. Healy pioneered the psychological study and treatment of the individual delinquent. Treatment was designed to help the individual to deal with aspects of his environment by encouraging him to reach out and by helping him in concrete ways to take advantage of existing educational, recreational, and vocational opportunities; that is, the social workers of that day (pre-World War I) went out and located troubled people. The very going out implied that the major locus of difficulty was not in something that the client carried around in his head but that existed in the conditions under which that client or that patient lived.

The Social Context of the Child Guidance Clinic

The year 1912 was the beginning of the end of the era of reform. A lot of the reforms of that day were associated with the Progressive Party, which, by 1914, had fallen apart. A great many reformers had participated in the pacifist movement, and consequently, suffered damaged reputations. During World War I, the war effort and patriotism dominated public opinion. Concern for problems of the poor, the working man, the women, children, the immigrant, the slum, and political and industrial-social reform was lost.

In the postwar period from 1920 until 1930, liberals and reformers were without influence or power. The Bolshevik Revolution had sparked a "Red Scare" that discouraged criticism of America and its institutions. During that period the businessman, the millionaire—Lindbergh, Babe Ruth, and even an Al Capone— could capture public attention and admiration because that was the era when success was admired, and success was viewed as a matter of individual effort.

The period of the 1920s was viewed as the best of all possible worlds. If you failed then, it was simply that you were inadequate to take advantage of that "best of all possible worlds." That was during the time that pop psychologist Coué swept the nation with his catch phrase, "Every day in every way I am getting better and better." The problem in the 1920s was to make the self better. In the pre-World War I era, the problem was to make the world better. Those are two vastly different orientations.

Industrial development and the war had led to a change in the relationships between the sexes. Participation by women in the labor force had steadily increased, and in 1920 the Nineteenth Amendment was passed, assuring women the right to vote. Changes in sexual behavior occurred. The virtues of premarital chastity and marital fidelity were challenged. The mass media purveyed the sexual theme and the theme of scientific human relations. It was in this period that psychoanalysis, emphasizing individual psychodynamics, took hold in the United States, providing an intellectual and scientific rationale for the changes that were taking place.

And parental thinking about how you raise your children in this world was affected. The question became how does one raise children in a world whose standards are markedly different from the standards of one's youth?

It was during this period of ferment that the child guidance clinic with its emphasis on scientific expertise in an area of grave concern took hold, and it flourished.

The Beginning Context

The Commonwealth Fund was established in 1918 in the pattern of philanthropy that was developed by those who had made their fortunes during the industrial and economic growth followiing the Civil War. That its first program focused on the prevention of delinquency reveals that it was planned on premises which reflected the climate of social reform of the pre-World War I era. The advisory committee that drew up the plans for the new program very clearly and explicitly stated that unresponsive and poorly trained teachers and school authorities, inadequate child welfare agencies, institutions for the retarded, detention and reform schools, insufficient recreational facilities, child labor, and inadequately trained probation officers in the juvenile court all contributed to causing juvenile delinquency by failing to observe youth adequately.

The conference report included a statement that existing social agencies needed to be carefully evaluated and needed to change if delinquency was to be prevented. In other words, their entire focus was not on the characteristics of delinquent youth but on the characteristics of social agencies that were serving youth. It was also obvious that the model of treating the sick who would come to the clinic for help was totally inadequate to the task of serving a community.

In 1922 a pilot project was swamped upon opening its doors. The planners knew immediately that if a service was provided for individuals then the needs of even a small community could not be met. The experience indicated it was necessary to develop strategies other than direct service to individuals.

The original goal of these clinics, as laid out in their plans, was to use mental hygiene personnel as consultants to workers in community agencies to help those workers deal more effectively with the children in their care. There was clear recognition of the need to develop indirect methods of treatment and ways of influencing aspects of the social environment if need was to be met. Within a decade, indeed almost from the establishment of the first of these clinics in the early 1920s, that goal of developing indirect methods was lost. Clinics chose to work with the individual rather than to work with the social structure.

Given the knowledge of the immense demand for service and the impossibility of meeting the demand by individual treatment, why did the clinics embrace the methods and doctrines of psychoanalysis, which focus on the individual? Why did they not seek to develop an applied sociology instead?

Forces Making for Change

The conservative tone of the 1920s favored an emphasis on individual responsibility instead of institutional responsibility. Reformers were out of favor and out of style. Trainers of psychiatrists and social workers in the mid-1920s complained that it was difficult to interest the young workers in the problems of consultation, community relations, and organization. They seemed to be interested in concepts of individual psychodynamics, not in institutional reform or institutional change. The older symbols of change were now stale and could no longer develop an emotional response in those who were coming into the field.

Social Work and Child Guidance

Child guidance clinics fall more in the domain of professional social work than any other field. The clinics originally included the three professions. The social worker was to relate to social agencies, the psychologist to relate to the schools and to give the intelligence tests that were popularized during World War I, and the psychiatrists were there to diagnose the disturbance and make recommendations for treatment. But social workers came to dominate the clinic, in numbers, if not in status.

Social work had originally been carried out by volunteers, but by 1919 there were already 17 professional schools of social work in the United States. Very early social workers were predominantly upper-class women engaged in charitable, humanitarian activities. When social work became an occupation, the pioneers were still upper-class, college-educated women who were seeking a new meaning for their own lives by finding a place in the changing society. Those first social workers were the first generation of young women for whom higher education had become a reality.

Marginal people and minority group members tend to flow into new occupations and new professions rather than into established ones, because the barriers of tradition are less formidable. Many women entered the new field of social work with the very conscious aim of attaining professional status. While there was pressure for professional standing from Smith, Vassar, Wellesley, and Radcliffe graduates, the pressure was even greater when those entering sought social and economic advancement through their profession.

Just as social work was striving toward professional standing, Abraham Flexner in 1915 concluded that social work lacked a communicable body of knowledge and a method that would be taught in schools, two of the characteristics of professions. Shortly after Flexner's address, Mary Richmond published *Social Diagnosis*, a comprehensive text on social casework methodology.

World War I produced another strong impetus toward the development of case work with the individual. Psychiatric social work began with the need to train workers to help treat the large number of neuropsychiatric casualties ("shell shock") that were produced by the war. *He* was the patient, not the society that produced the war.

Psychoanalysis and Social Work

Professionalization of the social work field had profound consequences for child guidance practice. Child guidance clinics were intended to serve a delinquent or a low-income population. Less than one-third of clinic cases overall came from middle- or upper-income groups. By 1948 those proportions had reversed. About 60 percent of referrals to privately supported clinics came from the upper-income population and that trend probably accelerated at least into the early 1960s.

This change in population requires some explanation since self-referred, middle-class cases, now considered most desirable, were originally seen as expensive to handle and as diverting effort from the community agencies' attempts to do a better job with the children that they already treated. Because social workers dealt with self-referred parents and particularly because they were influenced by psychoanalytic thinking, they focused more on the parent–child relationship, discovering that many parents wanted help for themselves. Clinics imposed a requirement that parents participate in the work of the clinic if their children were to be accepted for service. By 1930, the service became therapy for mothers by social workers and the social work literature increasingly focused on psychotherapy.

That change in the nature of service took place despite clear evidence that the earlier methods of social treatment and environmental manipulations had been effective. The change persisted despite evidence that the new form of treatment may have been inferior to the old in terms of improvement rates.

In the 1920s, social workers needed a professional method to achieve professional status. The method they relied upon was psychoanalytic casework. It is a reasonable assumption that the parent who brought the child to the clinic was more likely to speak the social worker's language, more likely to be from a background similar to the social worker, and more likely to share the social worker's life-style. It is reasonable to assume that such a client would not only be seen as more desirable but may have responded better to the interview technique that was used by the social worker. Over time, the approach would have favored one group—effectively screening out lower-income individuals who do not as a rule respond well to a talking treatment. It is also reasonable that the upwardly mobile social worker would have felt greater status in serving a more prestigious social class.

Over a period of years, the population of children and the type of problems that were seen in the clinics also changed. The clinic tended to deal with children whose difficulties were less severe or of recent origin. What is most paradoxical about this situation is that the professional mental health clinic accepted the easiest cases and left the community agencies, who were presumably staffed with the less well-trained people, with the more difficult problems. Over time, this situation reduced their consultative contacts with other agencies as well.

The Decade of the 1960s

Our thesis states that the conception of the mental health problem and the form of help that develops at any point in time is shaped by and will reflect general social conditions. During reform periods, the dominant philosophy seems to be one that emphasizes the spark of the divine in man. The social environment out there is seen as at fault. During conservative periods, the social world will be viewed as the best of all possible worlds, and individuals who have difficulty in living in a good social world will be viewed as sick. The form of help becomes one of removing the individual from the social setting, attempting to change him in some way, and then reintroducing him into the same setting.

In the early 1960s, during the Kennedy reform era, we tried to change the schools in some way, so that the urban poor would have better education. In the late 1960s, the Shockley-Jensen position, which asserted a genetically determined intelligence advantage of whites over blacks, attained prominence. What we saw was a shift to a much more politically conservative stance that seemed to say we are going to stop changing social institutions. Then we began to see the urban poor as inherently inferior. In the Kennedy reform period beginning in the early 1960s we had a focus on the problem out there in the social environment.

Some Speculations

Our own speculation is that the reforms that began in the 1960s were incomplete and were aborted by the Vietnam War. Our guess is that, barring the worsening of the energy crisis, in 5 or 10 years we will see the reemergence of reform as resources become available. We hope we will be more ready for it when the time comes, both conceptually and in terms of remembering our recent experiences.

The politician must be able to endure contradictions over a long period of time and not lose the will to resolve them. He cannot ignore either horn of a dilemma. Unions cannot be brushed off, nor can the obvious need for community-based services be casually dismissed. In his presentation of the deliberations involved in a new mental health bill for Pennsylvania, State Senator Louis Coppersmith, Chairman of the Committee on Health and Welfare, makes us experience the contrary forces shaping the legislation. We gain a sense of the vision and strength of character required to prevent too hasty a solution to a focal problem, involuntary commitment.

Chapter 3

THE POLITICS AND ECONOMICS OF HUMAN SERVICES AS SEEN FROM THE STATE LEGISLATOR'S VIEWPOINT

W. Louis Coppersmith

The Issue of Commitment

In past years, some of us have spoken of the remedy of three great areas of need in previously existing human service delivery systems: the absence of confidentiality, the absence of a patient advocacy service, and the existence of peonage. A fourth emerging issue is the very important area of voluntary and involuntary commitment. This is an area of great controversy now because of a Mental Health bill before my senate committee. The Pennsylvania 1966 Mental Health Act, in setting the standard of what constitutes a mental illness, and enabling someone to be involuntarily committed, is a very general statement. It says that anyone who is abnormal is suffering from a type of mental illness. The law must be interpreted by 67 different counties. In Pittsburgh, for instance, a person cannot be committed involuntarily unless, because of his illness, he has done something that would constitute a criminal act. This is a ridiculous formulation. Allegheny County's Judge Lowe, whom I have a great deal of respect for, justifies the involuntary commitments on the theory that if these persons have committed a criminal act, they could be involuntarily committed to a prison for the criminal act. So it is not a violation of his theory, then, if they are involuntarily committed to a hospital because they have committed this act; their civil liberties have not been violated in a way that affronts his conscience.

But if a person is mentally ill and is threatening to the community, I do not think that person should be committed while another person who is mentally ill but not posing a threat should not be committed, even though both may need the involuntary commitment to the same extent. It makes no medical sense to adopt that rationalization. In Philadelphia, you cannot be involuntarily committed unless you have threatened harm to another or yourself. Again, that is, in my opinion, too extreme a formulation, because what happens really is when you get too difficult a test for involuntary commitment, you must make perjurers out of the family. They could say, "Sure, he threatened to commit suicide," and on that basis the person is committed.

This involuntary commitment is really the heart of the controversy over the mental health bill. The ACLU and certain psychiatrists feel that no one should be involuntarily committed. If one is going to commit suicide, then that is their right. They have a right to refuse treatment; no one should be put in the hospital for care and treatment if they do not want it.

I always cite the classic case where a derelict is sitting on a park bench when it's 10 degrees below zero and is committing no crime. He does not want to move, and if he is left there for three hours, the man will freeze to death. I ask the people who are against any kind of involuntary commitment whether to preserve his civil rights and let him freeze to death, or violate his civil rights and take him to the hospital and save his life. I never get a direct answer to that question. It is too cruel to say you'd let the person freeze to death in the park rather than take him to the hospital against his will. This is the fatal fallacy of the people who are against any type of involuntary commitment.

Many older people become depressed and don't feed or care for themselves. They don't want to leave their home. They will waste away and die unless there is some kind of intervention. That is the fatal fallacy of the people who are against any type of involuntary commitment.

On the other side, you have the argument which has been advanced at my committee hearings on this bill, quite seriously, that there are many situations where the family finds it difficult or intolerable to have an individual to continue among it. In order to make it easy for the rest of the family, we should commit the patient even though he may not need treatment and it may not be beneficial to him. If he continues to live outside a hospital he can maintain himself and is not a danger to others. We are getting requests that people who have bizarre or manic behavior should be committed. This, then, the definition of what should allow commitment, is one of the key areas in which we are getting the flak with this bill.

The committee and I have come up with a formulation that a person who threatens serious bodily harm to hiimself or another within a limited period of time can be committed. He could be committed where it is probable that within a 30-day period, death, injury, or debilitation will occur. This covers the person in a deep depression who is not caring for himself, and it covers a person who threatens to commit suicide or harm to another. However, at present, we do not have in the bill a stipulation that bizarre or manic behavior will permit commitment. My own feeling is what's one person's bizarre or manic behavior is another person's eccentricity. And if my son wants to wear flowing robes and a long beard and live in that manner, unless he is not able to feed himself or maintain certain minimal functions properly, so long as he is not a danger to others or to himself, he should not be stopped from doing that. However, we are getting a great deal of pressure from psychiatrists associated with the state hospital institution who feel that there should be this right of intervention. There are many times that people who are manic will dissipate their estate, and there's nothing that can be done. It is very difficult to come up with a formulation that will differentiate between behavior that is true mental illness or eccentricity.

The legislature will have to decide where the greatest evil will come from. If we put in bizarre and manic behavior, will that impinge on the civil rights of people who are just different but really are not mentally ill? And if we don't put in the bizarre and manic behavior provision allowing involuntary commitment for that reason, then will we have people who should be treated and as a result will dissipate their estates and harm the families? It is a balancing of interests and there is no clear-cut decision one way or the other. This is one of the basic areas in which the committee's going to have to make a decision.

In the background on how broad to make this standard is a basic political fight that is going on right now in the state of Pennsylvania. California, which has adopted a policy of eliminating state mental institutions, has a population of about 7,000 in the state mental institutions out of a state population of 21 million. Perhaps

California has cut back too far, because there are cases where people who have been removed from the institutions who had not been able to make it, and who have great difficulties in life outside the institution. Pennsylvania, however, has a population of 17,000 in the state mental health institutions out of an overall population of 12 million. On a per capita basis, Pennsylvania has a much higher population in its state mental institutions than California.

Studies show that if a person is kept in a mental institution for two years, his chance of being able to live outside the institution is 6 out of 100. The difficulties caused by being in a mental institution for a prolonged period of time might be worse than those that caused their original admission. And think about what life would be like if you were in a mental institution day after day, week after week, year after year; perhaps with a staff that is not too feeling or considerate with others who have their own problems. Think of the problems it would cause to people who are normal to start out with, who are sensitive, and who are forced to live like that—with really not much hope for the future. You can see why this figure of 6 percent would be a valid one.

However, the employees of the mental hospitals in Pennsylvania are organized and have a union. Their basic goal is to preserve the job of each and every one of those employees. A policy to phase out these institutions runs counter to that goal.

Again, you have to understand that the county mental health program in Pennsylvania is not working as effectively or as efficiently as it should. They do not have adequate systems really to get information from each county as to the number of patients they serve and the cost per different type of service. In many areas there are weak mental health programs, and in some areas they are nonexistent. If patients are moved out of the mental hospitals, then supportive services must be in the local communities. In the last 10 years the cost of maintaining patients in a state institution has quadrupled. The number of patients has been halved, and the cost has doubled. The legislature is willing to appropriate only a limited amount of money for mental health institutions. And you have a question of establishing your priorities. You cannot continue to maintain existing populations in the mental institutions with rapidly spiraling costs, and, at the same time, have enough money to establish adequate county mental health services. Priorities have to be established. Can you find the money to strengthen the county mental health services unless you start cutting back on the state facilities? The argument used by those who do not want to cut back the state hospitals is that these patients are being dumped into the cities and areas where there are no services for them, and they will just be in a terrible situation. And this, quite possibly, is true. At the same time, if we keep the people in the mental hospitals, there will not be enough money to strengthen the county mental health programs as they should be strengthened.

Inevitably, when a person is discharged from a mental hospital, even if the local supportive services are adequate, there is no guarantee that he will be living a pleasant or a desirable life. As a practical matter, we have to do the best we can in the situation and "play the percentages." The percentages in Pennsylvania are to cut back on the number of patients in the state mental hospitals as much as possible. After all, the percentages are against you if you keep them in the mental hospitals. They are not going to get better. They are not going to be able to make it in society. The cost of maintaining them drains away money from other areas where the same money can benefit much larger numbers of people. What is going to benefit the most people over the longest period of time and, on balance, will create the least human suffering?

Isn't that a fair way to pose a question of what we have to do? That is why, in my opinion, we have to adopt some kind of policy that will result in a phasing out of the mental institutions in Pennsylvania and into the strengthening of the community mental health services. We cannot spend too much money on the limited number of people in institutions, while at the same time ignoring the thousands of people who do not belong in mental institutions, and, at the same time, lead a dreary and a terrible life because they are not getting adequate medical and other assistance in order for them to cope with the problems of modern life. One must understand that life for hundreds of thousands of people is very dreary and shabby because we are unable to provide a more efficient and imaginative community mental health service that would enable them to function better.

Of Politics and Economics

Those people who want to maintain the existing level of population (or near it) in the state mental institutions are seeking to have as broad a definition as possible for involuntary commitment, because this will enable the population to exist at the present levels. And those who are opposed to the present system want a very narrow definition.

The New Mental Health Bill

Within a couple of months we are going to be putting in a new bill, which will define policy for the state mental institutions. The bill covers confidentiality, commitment, a pilot program for the patient advocacy, and also the peonage question. I have tried to take the question of what the future of the state institutions will be out of this bill, which if you stop to think about it, with the exception of the scope of the provision concerning what will permit involuntary commitment, has nothing to do with the future of the state mental institutions.

However, people feel that this bill is but the stalking horse for a plan to phase out the state mental health institutions. As a result, we are involved in a terrible controversy with AFSCME, the AFL-CIO, and those psychiatrists and social service workers who have associations with the state hospitals. The degree of their opposition is quite astounding. In fact, they put out a letter that deliberately misrepresented the bill in its provisions. You would expect them at least to start out with the basic correct facts and perhaps draw different conclusions but not to try to distort the facts in order to support prearranged ideas. That is not a scientific way to do your work.

We must do something because the commitment provisions of the existing Mental Health Act are unconstitutional under recent decisions. In this bill, we have a little different procedure on the commitment procedures that I think is more in accord with reality. Right now, as I've mentioned before, in most cases to get someone involuntarily committed you have to perjure yourself. You have to say that they committed a crime or they threatened to commit suicide. And any law that requires perjury is a bad law in my opinion.

I started out with the premise that you have to have some kind of involuntary commitment. If a person is creating a terrible strain in the family at all hours of day and night you have terrible pressures on a family, so that they will do anything to get the person out; and it doesn't matter what kind of law you have. If you don't have an involuntary commitment law, the family will have them arrested. So to realize that society requires an effective kind of crisis intervention we have a provision that any doctor, upon stating that a person is severely mentally ill or severely mentally disabled, can get a person committed for up to 72 hours in a hospital. This is much easier than presently exists in many areas.

However, the real danger with involuntary commitments is once they start, they go on indefinitely. So we have a structure where we have a low threshold. Then after a person is in 72 hours, we require a hearing in the hospital before a mental health professional where the patient has the right to have counsel, and it has to be shown there that this person needs further involuntary commitment. The treatment has to start within two hours after he is involuntarily committed. A tape recording is kept to show the continued necessity of treatment for a period of no longer than 20 days.

If there should be a determination that treatment is needed after 20 days, then we require a court hearing, where all the due process safeguards are present, and a judge has to decide if there should be a further commitment of 90 days. A full-dress court hearing again has to decide for a one year commitment, which we think will be, at least if the judge is proper, an adequate safeguard.

So we start off the low threshold and we make it more and more difficult to keep the person in if he is involuntarily committed. To me, that was a procedure that was really more in tune with our needs, because the present law made it very difficult to get someone in, but once they were in, it was not too hard to keep them in. I think you have to have a situation where it's not that hard to get someone in, but then once they're in and the crisis is averted, it becomes extremely hard to keep them in. We've been meeting with psychiatrists and trying to work out something that is to their liking. Of course, the psychiatrists (most of them anyhow) feel that the definition for involuntary commitment should be quite broad. This is understandable since they feel that they understand the problems perhaps better than the lawyers or the legislators, and they should be allowed to decide what's best.

It was very interesting to hear some of the mental health professionals who felt that they knew what was best for everybody. But many of them feel that they should be given the broadest possible power to determine if someone needs treatment. If someone does not need treatment—even if they're not a threat to themselves or others—a lot of mental health professionals feel that maybe they'll like life a little better if they get treatment. Me, I don't agree with that philosophy. I think just like if I have a chronic ailment and I don't want treatment, as long as I'm not a threat to myself or others, why do I have to have treatment? This is a libertarian concept which, as I said before, many mental health professionals aren't quite in sympathy with.

The Genesis of the New Mental Health Bill

The genesis of Senate Bill 1239 came out of the need for a new mental health bill because much of the 1966 MHMR Act was unconstitutional on commitment procedures. The new bill would make changes in the county set-up and would be designed to phase out the state institutions. The original draft presented by the Department of Public Welfare did deal with the phasing out of the state institutions and did not have the type of commitment procedure I've discussed—you know, the threshold and then making it more difficult to keep people in. They presented it to me and my committee and I worked on it. We came up with the involuntary commitment procedures I've outlined. We also came up with the pilot programs for the patient-advocacy service. The committee, the chairman (myself), and Senator Scales made quite a number of extensive changes in the draft.

We dealt with the southeastern Pennsylvania group that works on mental health problems and got their input into this. We then submitted it to the Pennsylvania Psychiatric Association, and conducted hearings across the state. The subcommittee had maybe six hearings and the full committees had three hearings on this proposal, seeking to get input from all of those involved, including the Pennsylvania Psychiatric Association and the AFL-CIO. The psychiatric association was afraid that we were undermining the power of the psychiatrists. They wanted broader involuntary commitment procedures. They really had a number of very practical suggestions, a lot of which we have adopted. Their input is in the bill to a very great extent, and we tried to adopt their suggestions whenever we could.

The concern of the AFL-CIO really basically boils down to jobs in the mental health system, although, of course, they would never say that; but when you strip away the verbiage and baloney, it's jobs. The social workers are concerned about not having too severe a cutback in the state mental health institutions and are also concerned about jobs.

The Pennsylvania Mental Health Association has been in the forefront of seeking legislation to improve the laws on the mentally ill and getting adequate funding for the hospitals and working toward eliminating the state hospitals. Unfortunately in this whole business, they were split up among themselves by those who were opposed to any involuntary commitment and those who favored some type of involuntary commitment. They were so split up that they have been unable to afford to the committee any positive detailed statement as to what they would like in the bill. It's tragic, really, that on a doctrinaire issue that they would divide themselves so that they could not effectively participate in really what may be the most important legislation in this area for many years.

Originally, we were going to have the bill include a provision for the retarded along with the mentally ill. The Pennsylvania Association of Retarded Citizens (PARC) wanted a separate bill, because they felt that the mentally ill are always considered before the retarded. So they wanted their own bill, and we agreed. However, now we have a situation where the same opponents of phasing out the mental institutions are opposed to phasing out the institutions for the retarded. PARC is very strongly for phasing out the institutions for the retarded and for having community set-ups. So the opponents of PARC and of the policy we're trying to establish for the mentally ill are the same. But PARC, because of its doctrinaire hang-ups, doesn't want to be associated with the mentally ill. So the proponents of phasing out the institutions are divided, while the proponents of keeping the institutions are united. These problems hamper us greatly in trying to change the direction in regard to the mental institutions for the retarded. And of course, the Welfare Department favors the phasing out of the institutions.

A Favorable Outcome?

Unfortunately, I really don't think the legislature addresses itself to the question of the appropriations and the priorities. It is very difficult to establish a priority here, because you're putting someone ahead of someone else and the person who's put behind is upset. And it means controversy. And, as a result, you never do establish priorities. This has been one of the problems in the mental health field. People are saying that we have to have better treatment in our state mental institutions and we have to take care of the patients. But at the same time, money spent on mental health institutions means that community programs are going to be short-changed. There's not enough money to do both. But people want to put a little more money in the community programs and in the institutions; the legislature just won't deal with a difficult question like establishing priorities unless they're forced to.

People don't realize that there is a contradiction here; that, in the long run, urging more money for the mental institutions might not be the most humane or the best thing to do simply because these institutions are generally harmful to people.

The commitment procedures are, of course, in shambles because of court decisions. The county mental health programs are extremely spotty. In a few areas they are good, in some areas they are nonexistent, and in some areas they are very poor. They have no basis for controlling and getting adequate information the way they should. There is no correlation between the programs and the institutions. They are trying to perform some kind of concerted action, but there's really no comprehensive plan that's being developed now or that's being implemented. This is really my basic indictment of the whole set-up.

There is a task force that went into the goals of our MHMR program and that had a completely different appproach than I have. Pennsylvania Mental Health was very active in this task force. Their theory was to establish a program known as *Outreach*, manned 24 hours a day with a mental health professional, who would examine a person before he could be involuntarily committed. It was an expensive system to get state intervention before anyone could be involuntarily committed. This system was to seek out peop,e who were mentally ill and get them treatment.

I don't agree with this policy at all; this sounds like Big Brother. In Russia, if a person disagrees politically, he is put in an insane asylum. To me this has dangerous connotations that the state should actively be seeking out people who are mentally ill, and they are going to help them. If a person wants help, you have to have a system to give him help. And they can be encouraged. But you have to be careful that you are not too insistent or aggressive in this area. I think you can never forget the implicit dangers to civil liberty of such a program, and I think our policy should be to eliminate the institutions as much as possible and to have the adequate facilities in the community. Because, if they are there, they are used, as is shown by those programs that are working well.

Looking at mental health from the legal, historical, or moral point of view must be supplemented by a structural view of the state's commitment to the mental hospital as the main instrument for dealing with mental disorders. Secretary Beach presents us with a problem that would tax the most clever group of systems analysts. The facets of the problem include the patients, the staff, the buildings, the vast lands, the economic impact on the community, the unprepared family of the released long-term patients, pressures of budget and fiscal demand, determination of quality of care, safety codes, competition for dollars, and so on. Community-based services are handling a far greater proportion of the patient population at a fraction of the state hospital's budget. The community based services exist due to the initiative and funding support of the federal government. When funding is phased out, the state might miss the opportunity of saving millions of bond and tax dollars. Which way will the state go?

Chapter 4

DEINSTITUTIONALIZING THE GENERAL MENTAL HEALTH DELIVERY SYSTEM

William B. Beach, Jr.

Many states have been going through the difficult problem of deinstitutionalizing or reducing and eliminating the need for hospitalization of the mentally ill in the state mental hospitals. The problems are complex, and this can be readily seen as one pays attention to the resistances and concerns that are expressed as soon as there is any public discussion relating to the potential closings or eliminating large numbers of staff at state mental hospitals. Two states can be used easily as examples in this area: California, which has had many years of experience in moving from institutional to community programs, and Pennsylvania which has a very far advanced community mental health program that is having a major impact on the utilization of state hospitals. Although both states emphasize a community program based on county government being the recipient of state funds, there are many differences between the two states.

The Initial Problems: A Comparison

Pennsylvania is a state that is not growing in population, whereas for several years the population of California has expanded rapidly. This rapid growth in itself produces problems in the planning and development of services. In the California situation, they are not only trying to reorganize what is already there, but also it is becoming necessary to build in all of the demands of the increasing population.

Both state legislatures have two houses: Pennsylvania has a legislature composed of 253 members as compared to California's 120 members. The 120 legislators in California serve 20 million people in a state that extends 1000 miles from Oregon to Mexico. The 253 legislators in Pennsylvania serve about 12 million people and therefore are closer and more involved with the mental health institutions that are in their areas. This is emphasized even more by the fact that California had only 10 hospitals for the mentally ill compared to 19 in Pennsylvania. When a facility is in the legislator's district, there is much more personal advocacy in the legislature and a direct concern with what is happening to the constituency.

In California, the Short Doyle community mental health program began in 1957. The impact on the state mental hospitals became noticeable when payment for involuntary mental health care provided locally was authorized and, most especially, in 1969 when new legislation combined the state and community programs. Currently, the state hospital in California provides services to counties they serve according to an approved plan whereby the state hospital becomes "an extension" of the community program.

In California, the state hospitals for many years have been under central administration with uniform policies and procedures governing their operation; for many years, hospitals in Pennsylvania were autonomous facilities governed by administrative boards of trustees, with each institution going independently to the legislature for its budget. It was not until recent years that they came under central direction, and the boards of trustees became advisory. As a result of years of independent approach, each hospital is often very different from others. At one time, they also were dependent on patient labor for operation and maintenance and had large farming operations that helped to support the operation of the institution. As traditions developed and became established over decades of such operation, changes in direction and new concepts of care and treatment can have a great impact upon personnel. In Pennsylvania, most of the institutions were built in rural areas with small communities developing around them. They became the principle economic and employment resource for the area served. Buildings were added over the years so that each hospital had a mixture of new buildings and old unsafe buildings. As an example, one hospital had three main buildings: one brand new building was dedicated two years ago; a second building was opened 20 years ago; and a third building which housed most of the patients opened 114 years ago. One-half of the buildings in the Pennsylvania mental hospital system are over 50 years of age; a third, over 80 years of age. This means that the cost of maintenance, upkeep, and repairs can be expensive. Statistics relative to admissions and resident population and personnel in the Pennsylvania facilities can also give some idea of the trends that have been developing.

Year	Admissions	Resident Population June 30th	Personnel
1965	16,793	35,514	19,617
1969	13,992	28,330	16,912
1974	8,050	18,000	15,900

As shown by these figures, there has been a marked decrease in the number of admissions, a decrease in the number of patients in the hospital, and an increase in staff–patient ratios over 1965, although there is now beginning to be some decline in staff. Here again, however, statistics need to be eveluted carefully, because with 20 different institutions the situation takes on a different appearance. For example, there are hospitals in which the decline in patients has been large while the numbers of staff has remained about the same, but the classification of staff is not appropriate to the needs of the hospital. For example, many hospitals are very short on numbers of trained professionals such as psychiatric nurses, licensed practical nurses, and physicians, whereas another hospital of the same size in a metropolitan area will have a very different staffing pattern for the same population.

Staffing patterns were not developed over the years to determine what kinds of staff a facility would need to have, nor were any staffing ratios established. For example, there was no determination on how many psychiatrists, social workers, rehabilitation workers, gardeners, farmers, butchers, etc., a hospital should have for a given population with certain characteristics. Superintendents were given positions that they could fill in any way they wanted, and they took opportunities as they occurred. If they had an opportunity to hire a psychiatrist, they could select a "vacant position" and hire a psychiatrist. If, on the other hand, they had the opportunity to hire a clerk or a butcher or a groundskeeper which they felt that they needed at that point, they could use that same vacant position to do that. This meant that a very different staffing pattern developed for each hospital over the years. Philadelphia State Hospital is an example where there were 6200 patients in 1965 compared to 1400 patients currently, and they are decreasing at about the rate of 300 to 400 patients a year. Coinciding with that drop, however, there has not been a drop in total staff in the same proportions, so that, currently, there are approximately 1880 staff for 1400 patients. It may seem rather well off in the way of staffing, but this is not totally true; the hospital is desperately short of nursing and housekeeping staff. On the other hand, there are large numbers of clerical staff, full-time chaplains, etc. The proportions of staff are wrong.

There are other reasons that have contributed to this over a period of time. When money has gotten tight, vacant jobs are not allowed to be filled, which further saves money. Usually vacancies occur most often in the professional staff concerned with the treatment of patients, while the basic support personnel such as clerical, groundskeepers, farmers, etc., tend to stay on. As a result, those positions do not get abolished, and over a period of time, the imbalance increases. These are just some of the reasons that one cannot look at an individual institution in isolation from the whole system, anymore than you can look at the whole system without looking at what goes on with respect to each individual institution.

Another problem in the Pennsylvania system relates to the geriatric population. The need for community resources for this group is considerable, and nursing home development has been far behind what it is required to be. Mayview Hospital, near Pittsburgh, with 1880 patients has the following age categories: 13 patients under the age of 21; 888 patients aged 21 to 64; and 849 patients or approximately 50 percent of the population, age 65 or over. Some of these patients have been there for many years, and have grown old in the hospital; the community resources are not there to receive them, and the likelihood of relocation is slim. For the state system as a whole, about 36 percent of the hospital population is over 65.

The future of the state employee is another problem. Some years ago jobs were filled by patronage and were often political appointments. Every time there was a change in administration people would leave and new people were appointed; that, fortunately, changed when civil service came into being. In addition, most state employees are in a union. This includes in the Pennsylvania system physicians who are not in administrative roles. Each union has bargaining rights, and these relate to overtime, grievances, salaries, fringe benefits, etc. The future of the employee becomes extremely important when you plan in relation to a declining population in the mental hospital.

Even though the population has gone down, cost of care has gone up considerably because of inflation, improved care, and increased employee benefits. The legislature, at times, has difficulty understanding why the budget grows in both the community and the hospital programs when the hospital population and admissions are declining. When the method of reducing hospital costs relates to closing some of the institutions, consolidating some, eliminating jobs, and laying off employees many problems occur. Some legislators will say this should be done, but will not touch the one in their area. Their constituents are these employees whose jobs are threatened. These employees have entered a system thinking they had a lifetime career. Many have had many years of services, the fringe benefits have improved, the retirement benefits are good, and one does not just pull a job away from somebody and destroy everything that he has been working for, especially when the state has probably recruited him for the system.

What do you do when somebody has been in the system and has 10 or 15 years of service? The answer is usually not to touch them but to abolish vacant positions as they occur. But as already indicated, the problems are many and also vacancies do not always occur in the right institutions in the right categories at the right time. Some of this is the same struggle that has gone on for several years in California. Actually, they have closed some of their facilities. The employees have demanded a legislative investigation and a deemphasis on pushing community programs any further because they felt that communities were not ready for it. It is true that, in many instances, the communities were not ready, and in metropolitan areas such as New York, Los Angeles, Pittsburgh, and Philadelphia, it appeared that former mental hospital patients were being warehoused in the community, instead of being taken care of adequately. In some instances, they seemed to be much better off when they were in hospitals. There was strong emphasis in the California program on reducing the number of admissions to the state hospitals and providing alternatives at that point, as well as moving people out of the hospital who were already there. However, adequate planning for services for those moving out of the hospitals was apparently lacking.

Comparing Costs

The costs of maintaining a mental hospital are many, and if one could find a way to shift the dollars from the hospital to the community, it would be most helpful. It currently takes about $20 million a year in new funds just to maintain the hospitals at the level they are at with nothing new added. This, on top of the previous year's budget, is due to inflation and other factors. The 1400 patients at Philadelphia State Hospital require a budget of $23 million. Compare this to the community mental health budget for the entire state, which is about $35 million for approximately 100,000 patients. Making a shift of dollars from one system to another is a tremendous undertaking. The constraints already mentioned make it extremely difficult. Of major importance with respect to the state employees working in the institutional setting, there is a need to look at ways in which some of these employees might be used in the community programs, even perhaps remaining on the state payroll while working under the supervision of the local program. In this way, benefits that they have accumulated through the years of service can be safeguarded, but this will not take care of more than a small proportion of the personnel.

Other considerations that have been discussed include retraining of personnel, early retirement with lump-sum settlements in lieu of salary for X number of years, and varieties of other procedures, none of them simple. In places like California, the movement of personnel to community programs is facilitated in that the civil service system of the state is linked to county civil service, so that if a person moves from the state system to the county system, or vice versa, he transfers with him all of his retirement benefits. It would also benefit not only employees but patients to use the expertise that many of those in the state hospital have. To lose that experience would be unfortunate. One of the areas in which the hospital employee is often most expert is in working with the long-term, chronic, mentally ill patient who has been in the hospital for many years. Ideally, as systems of care are developed in the community that require a protective living situation, along with adequate programs, those skilled in working with such patients in the mental hospital would be utilized in the community setting with this group.

Anticipating Change

There are also new changes occurring downstream that must be anticipated. Many of these changes are dependent on the federal activities related to funding and utilization review. Patterns of care are affected greatly through the mechanisms of federal funding of programs. What is going to happen with respect to continuing community mental health funding by the federal government is not known, nor is it known what will happen with national health insurance with Professional Service Review Organizations (PSRO) and Utilization Review requirements, with tighter controls and restrictions relating to Medicaid and Medicare, etc. Likewise, there is increasing coverage by third-party private insurance carriers for mental illness. As this coverage increases, people will have funds available to obtain hospitalization in their own local community, rather than relying on the state to pay for this service in a state hospital. However, there are still dilemmas involving patterns of funding from the federal government. For example, the funding of community mental health centers takes care of staffing and construction. This is quite a different approach from proposed national health insurance plans, which are insurance programs designed to pay for service rendered, rather than funding the facility and its staff. Unknowns exist with the Health Maintenance Organization (HMO) and with where this program will go and how the community mental health program will fit in with it. Obviously, the development of increased insurance coverage, whether by private carriers or through national health insurance, can have a marked impact on the utilization of state hospitals.

Other dimensions to the problem of deinstitutionalization have to do with the physical plant itself. Pennsylvania has some of the most prized herds of cattle in the state. These are expensive herds, and perhaps they could be sold, but again, with prevailing problems of inflation, perhaps they can be consolidated and used to help support the food needs of the hospital population. On the other hand, the requirements for this volume of food supply will decrease as the hospital population decreases. The land occupied by the hospitals is sizeable, and a question arises about the need for the huge acreages and to what use this acreage may be put. Should it be leased to others to farm? Should it be turned into park lands? Should it be turned into state college areas? Acreages of this sort cannot be allowed to grow wild. There is a need for maintenance and fire protection. Abandoned buildings become areas where people can get hurt and fires can be started. Demolition of unused huge structures of the type of brick and concrete construction that characterize many of the buildings is a very expensive proposition in itself. Perhaps some buildings in some areas could be adapted to other uses such as offices if the area is a metropolitan one. In most instances, they could not meet fire safety codes without a tremendous cost for renovation.

Planning Deinstitutionalization

To effect changes in the institution requires a massive effort on the part of all involved groups and individuals. Planning needs to involve the board of trustees of the hospital, the administration of the hospital, appropriate state personnel, the county mental health and mental retardation board, and the other agencies and groups in the community who are affected by any proposed changes. Through such a joint effort any proposed plan must be evaluated on its merits, and determination made on what is practical and feasible, and to see when, how, and what can be implemented or changed.

Several other states besides California and Pennsylvania have been facing this problem of declining admissions and populations. The State of Washington had three state mental hospitals. They closed one about four years ago; the second one is slated to be closed this summer, leaving one remaining. Massachusetts has closed one state hospital and has come out with a detailed study and plan calling for the closing of all mental hospitals in five years. It is expected that they will have to backtrack on that since the reactions have been considerable.

In summary, whenever one considers deinstitutionalizing a mental health delivery system, there are multiple facets that need to be given careful consideration. These include the welfare of the patients who are affected; the welfare of the employees who are often times long-time career persons with highly skilled and technical abilities; the utilization of vacant buildings and unused land that is created by closure or decrease in size; the economic impact upon the community in which the hospital is located; the reactions of families and relatives to a change regarding a patient whom they have felt was permanently situated in the hospital for the rest of his life; pressures of budget and fiscal demands, coupled with inflationary problems and the need to continue to assure quality program but at appropriate cost; the problem of renovation and keeping buildings in conformance with lift safety codes; the competition for the dollar to be used by other groups who are also in acute need of funds; the need to continue to expand community programs as rapidly as practical and finding the money to do this.

Obviously, these and other factors not listed require, not a unilateral or a single agency involvement, but multiple groups representing all of these interests; these need to be included in the overall planning, which should put the patient first and foremost. The patient is what the entire system is about and what it is for. Planning must give attention to maximizing available facilities, manpower, and dollars, and finding the right proportions. A plan must also have short-range goals and long-range goals which can be altered as circumstances and new knowledge is learned.

Lucille Robuck, humanitarian and reform-oriented administrator in Kentucky's criminal justice system, tells of the function of parole in the correctional process. Noting that most parolees return to the communities from where they came, Robuck asserts that communities would be well advised to shoulder major responsibility for a positive transition to life outside prison walls. She describes the cooperation of the parole system with Community Mental Health Centers, some of the obstacles to such cooperation and how they have been overcome.

Chapter 5

COMMUNITY MENTAL HEALTH SERVICES AND THE PAROLEE'S TRANSITION TO NORMAL LIFE

Lucille Robuck

I would like to begin by briefly discussing the attitudes of the various persons the defendant comes in contact with upon entering the criminal justice system, including the parole board. The offender's attitude toward the criminal justice system is often formed very early in life by the attitude of his parents and his peers. Often his attitude is negative, and, therefore, it is even more important that this negative attitude is not reinforced by his first contact with the system. The arresting officer who handles the arrest in a professional manner can make a lasting contribution to the offender's future attitude toward law enforcement officials. The commonwealth attorney who *prosecutes* rather than *persecutes* can leave the offender with a positive, rather than negative, view of the system. The sentencing judge who treats the defendant with dignity enhances the person's positive image of the system and can cause him to be much more receptive to the staff and the treatment programs provided by the instution where he is incarcerated.

If the institutional staff continues to reflect a positive, helpful attitude toward the incarcerated man, and if he is willing to work in order to help himself, the parole board he will eventually appear before must also reflect a professional attitude in order not to destroy all the efforts that have been directed toward the person up to that point. This does not mean he will necessarily be granted parole. It does mean, however, that he is entitled to a fair and impartial review by a competent board, acting in the best interest of the individual before them and the community. He should be treated with dignity, and the Kentucky Parole Board, of which I am Chairman, makes every effort to do just that.

The Structure of the Parole Board

We are very fortunate in Kentucky to have been provided with legislation that requires prospective members of the parole board to have certain professional standards, and they must be screened by a nonpartisan committee who recommends those qualified to the Governor who then fills existing vacancies from the approved lists of applicants. No more than three of the five members may have the same political party affiliation, which prevents allegations of political interference.

The parole board is a major phase in the cycle of criminal justice, and if it is a weak, indifferent, or just plain incompetent board, or if it operates as a political entity to be used or misused by the political structure of the state, then the whole correctional cycle breaks down. Another person who could be restored to a law-abiding life in the community has become a victim of a system he did not trust in the first place, and his negative attitudes are just reinforced.

I am not saying the parole board is *the* major phase, but it is a phase that cannot be ignored. If the person appearing before the board has met all the requirements normally expected for a successful parole candidate and is not considered a danger to the community or to himself, then it logically follows that he should be released on parole. If he faces a board who denies him parole because "he has not served enough time" or some other poor reason, then a gigantic step backward can be expected. If, however, the board members make an honest effort to evaluate his strengths and weaknesses and takes time to place stipulations on his parole that will help him upon his reentry into the community, the parolee can return to society with a positive approach, utilizing the resources in the commounity to assist him along the way.

The Comprehensive Care Center

I would like to elaborate today on just one of the community resources that the Kentucky Parole Board is now using in the reintegration process. There are federally funded Comprehensive Care Centers scattered throughout the United States to provide mental health services at a community level. We are very fortunate in Kentucky to have a network of these Comprehensive Care Centers that are located throughout the state. In July of 1972, the Parole Board, with the cooperation of the Kentucky Department of Mental Health, decided to take advantage of these centers for persons leaving the institution on parole status. If the Parole Board deemed that the services of the Comprehensive Care Center would be helpful to the parolee, then it was made a stipulation of his parole that he must have counseling with the local Comprehensive Care Center in his area and continue until such time as the staff at the Comprehensive Care Center felt he no longer was in need of their services.

It has long been recognized that many persons upon entering the institution had long-standing emotional disturbances which had gone undiagnosed or untreated prior to their incarceration. Much progress has been made during the past several years to provide services for these persons while incarcerated, but due to limitations in the size of professional staff and the reluctance of psychiatrists to work within the confines of a prison wall, very little long-term treatment could be provided except in the most severe cases.

Many inmates falling into the marginal group needing services have benefited from group therapy while incarcerated but obviously need supportive help upon release. Thus, the Parole Board sought to provide this type of professional help following their release on parole through referrals to the Comprehensive Care Centers in the community where they will be residing.

Problems in Inaugurating the Centers

A number of problems surfaced almost immediately upon the board's installation of this referral program. One of the major problems was to convince the inmate being released on parole that this was not a service for the "crazy." These services have been presented to the inmates as professional services provided to keep healthy people healthy and to assist them in the normal everyday problems they will face upon being integrated into the community. Many of the inmates also had marriage problems prior to incarceration and were obviously going to face them upon release. In those instances, marriage counseling was suggested, and they were encouraged to interest their wives or husbands in going with them. Budget problems are almost universal to an individual going back into society, and it was stressed that this was an area where their caseworker at the Comprehensive Care Center could assist.

For the persons who had a prior history of mental illness, the Parole Board took great efforts to explain to them that if they had pneumonia they would seek a medical doctor, and in instances of emotional disturbances, the wise man secured the help of a psychiatrist. Most of the severe cases had some understanding of this and had received prior treatment either before they came to the institution or while in the institution. They recognized the need for professional help, particularly if they were from an urban area where this type of help had been available for some time. The Parole Board found it most difficult to explain the benefits of outpatient treatment care to the natives of eastern Kentucky, who came from a culture where strong emphasis was placed upon a man's "maleness" being defined as one who could handle his own problems. The Parole Board still meets more resistance to referrals from this area than from persons in other areas of the state.

A second major problem encountered was to break down the distrust that seemed to exist between the staffs of the Comprehensive Care Centers and the parole officers who would be responsible for seeing that these referrals were carried out when the man returned to the community. In conversations with the Comprehensive Care staff, it surfaced that there was a general feeling the parole officers were "policemen" and were trying to catch the men doing something they should not and therefore, the Comprehensive Care staff was very reluctant to share information with the parole officers. The parole officers verbalized many feelings that indicated they distrusted the Comprehensive Care staff because they were "social workers" who condoned unacceptable behavior of the parolees and "looked down" upon the parole officers, who were only doing their job. This area of mutual distrust took quite some time to unravel and alleviate, but it is practically nonexistent at this time. Much assistance was provided in this area by the central office staffs of both Probation and Parole and the Bureau for Health Services working together. It was discovered that a much better working climate existed as the two staffs got to know each other on a personal basis and realized each could be mutually supporting in their assistance to the client. One method adopted to alleviate mistrust and assist in developing a common philosophy was a seminar held in th₄ Louisville area. The seminar included the area with the largest number of Comprehensive Care Centers and the largest number of referrals by the Parole Board. In addition to the technical knowledge obtained, the best side effect was the personal staff relationships that developed.

A third area of confusion arose from the very realistic problem of transportation to and from the Comprehensive Care Centers for those persons who lived in rather remote areas. This had gradually been alleviated as the Comprehensive Care Centers have provided mobile units which go into rural areas on a weekly basis.

The fourth area of concern was the effectiveness of the referrals to Comprehensive Care Centers. At the end of fiscal year 1972-1973, a list of the names of all persons referred to the Comprehensive Care Centers throughout the state was given to a central office staff member of the Bureau for Health Services, along with the names of the towns where these persons were paroled in an effort to determine how many of them had made contact with the Comprehensive Care Centers as directed by the Parole Board. This turned out to be a monumental task when it was discovered that the Bureau for Health Services kept their records by Social Security numbers of those referred. However, the task was finally accomplished by the staff of the Bureau for Health Services, despite the lack of information provided; and it was determined that in the Parole Board's first year of concentrated referrals that only 50 percent of those referred actually got to the Comprehensive Care Center. This, of course, was discouraging and reflected the lack of understanding on the part of some of the Probation and Parole Officers, both of the program and also the unavailability of the program to persons in remote areas. As explained earlier, both these problems later were solved to a great extent. Thus, the Parole Board took the attitude that we did not have a 50 percent failure rate but a 50 percent success rate because we had more persons now receiving counseling and treatment from an outside resource than we ever had before. At an annual meeting with all of the Probation and Parole staff from around the state during October, 1973, these statistics were presented by me as the Chairman of the Parole Board to the Probation and Parole Officer's staff. They were not criticized for their failure in 50 percent of the cases that had no contact but were further urged to visit the staff of their local Comprehensive Care Center and utilize their assistance in handling their caseload. It was also pointed out that statistics would be kept in the future in an effort to detemine what areas were meeting with the most success and utilizing the help available. This meeting turned out to be quite beneficial and reemphasized the importance of using community resources.

During July 1973, the Parole Board began getting the social security numbers of all men who were referred to Comprehensive Care and passing these along to the Bureau for Health Services in order that the results could be determined on a better basis. Again, complications arose as the Bureau for Health Services was at that time installing a new computer, and the Parole Board was asked to devise a questionnaire which could be computerized in order to obtain the desired information. This led to further problems when an effort was made to devise not only the number of contacts with the client but also the quality of contacts. This problem is still being worked on, and it will probably be several years before any valid statistical data can be retrieved concerning this matter. Despite all of the problems, it has been very encouraging to observe the distrust between two state agencies fade, and a concerted effort to work together in a congenial manner for the benefit of the people who receive the services blossom in its stead.

Many problems occur when new programs are initiated, and the extensive use of Comprehensive Care Centers for offender rehabilitation was no exception. The operation is ongoing, and problems are solved by close coordination at all levels between the affected agencies. The major problem that continues to exist is that of data development, storage, and retrieving. When satisfactorily solved, the data collected over a five-year testing period will prove invaluable in accurately evaluating the effectiveness of the program.

Effectiveness of the Kentucky Centers

Using data currently available, it is estimated that about 95 percent of parole referrals actually make contact with the Comprehensive Care Center during the early stages of their period of parole, and these contacts are producing a positive impact on the success rate of the affected parolees. This has proved exceptionally helpful to those individuals with emotional and alcohol problems. The success rate for this category of the parolee has increased by 20 to 30 percent since the initiation of the referral program.

Needless to say, I am very enthusiastic about the referral system I have just described. The Kentucky Parole Board utilizes a number of other community-based programs such as halfway houses, volunteers, Alcoholics Anonymous, and others. I am firmly convinced that as time goes on, and with the efforts of all persons connected with the criminal justice system, we can tap other resources in the community by letting them know of our need. After all, the incarcerated person is often the product of the community to which he will return, and it is only fitting that the persons in the community be asked to help in this return. By doing so, they not only offer a helping hand to a fellow citizen but make their community a safer place in which to reside.

Given that an institution is an instrument society produces to meet the community's needs, any given institution becomes problematic when it itself generates problems of a magnitude equal to these it is supposed to solve. Such is the case with mental hospitals. From his 40 years of experience with the state's attempt to address mental problems through large mental "hospitals," Mr. Dybwad presents a nightmare concocted of economic pressures, totally self-contained infernos, and the ingenious legal maneuvers required to end a reign of terror the mentally ill and retarded have experienced. Without the background presented here, right to education and treatment legislation is incomprehensible.

Chapter 6

THE LAW AND MENTAL HEALTH
IN COMMUNITY SERVICES

Gunnar Dybwad

For those with experience in community mental health, child psychiatry, and a typical child guidance clinic, what I will say about the obstacles that must be removed in order to bring mental health towards community programs, and the role law is playing in this at the present time, may seem totally strange. I want to point this out right away because, for people who are involved in child psychiatry, Pavlov, the physiologist and Pennhurst, Polk, Rice, and Willowbrook, institutions for the mentally retarded, are names they have never heard or are beyond their conception. And yet they are landmarks of the historical background of my perspective on the topic; there will be other people to fill out the mental health picture in other respects.

Definitions

The term *mental health* is used here. The problem is that mental *health* in this country is either used as a synonym for mental *illness*, or it is used in very broad general terms encompassing mental illness, such as *neuroses*, which, in the past, were not mental illnesses, mental retardation, drug addiction, alcoholism, etc. When we talk about mental health we are dealing with a rather peculiar term, and one that is really quite new in this country. The National Association for Mental Health has existed only since 1950; the National Institutes of Mental Health since the late 1940s. Previously, we had a National Committee on Mental Hygiene, which was created in 1909.

Mental health is used today as a very broad, all-embracing term in which the pathologic connotations are greatly diminished. As discussed in schools, mental health refers to general well-being of people, much in line with the World Health Organization's definition of health as "a state of complete physical, mental, and social well being, and not merely the absence of disease or infirmity" (1946).

Myths and Mindtraps: A Brief History

As I have suggested, other people have different perspectives on the history of mental health. A psychiatrist, for example, would discuss the history of mental health to explain why Sigmund Freud arrived at his theories. He would talk about things that are totally different from the things I want to mention very briefly. One of the surviving heritages of medieval times is demonism. The then scientific explanation for mental illness was that people were possessed by demons. This was not simply folklore; it was the accepted professional explanation. Part of the very strong opposition encountered now when we try to introduce a widening of community mental health goes back precisely to these medieval superstitions. And more recently the Soviet dictatorship has given us yet another orientation to mental health—that of the police state, of law and order, or constraint, coercion, deportation. In other words, mentally ill and mentally retarded persons, like other grossly deviant people, were moved out of society into the "appropriate facilities." (These differed from country to country, but in the United States the results were these large institutions we called mental hospitals or state schools.) In the course of a lawsuit before a federal judge, a group of assistant attorney generals, associate commissioners for the New York State Department of Mental Hygiene, and some staff on the institutions for the mentally retarded toured the Middlebrook institution in New York. Our attorneys (of course the attorneys for the plaintiffs who had brought the suit) led us into the building where one attorney, who knew more about the institution than the commissioners, said, "Open this door, please. We have the right under court to go anywhere." And the door was opened to a seclusion room, and behind the door was a young woman. The attorney asked the staff member how long this person had been in seclusion (solitary confinement). It had been seven years! There is no penal system in this country that would keep a person in seclusion for seven years. In the mental health system, people—without adjudication or any formalities—were brutalized, imprisoned; and maltreated in ways that beg description. This is merely institutional lawlessness playing its very important role. The history behind this lawlessness is crucial.

One historical element is the eugenic scare in the early twentieth century, which was a reinforcement for the policy of segregation. I was the lead-off witness in *Poplar vs Alabama*, Poplar being a low functioning resident of an institution for retardates. After some initial questions, the attorney asked me, "Would you then say that what was offered to these people was no more than custodial care?" And I said, "No." He was temporarily taken aback. And I pointed out that custody involves certainly a minimum of safe keeping, and nobody could possibly talk about safe keeping with the conditions in those institutions.

You might say the same thing about the Philadelphia jail. Any place that people are raped, almost under a kind of official sanction, hardly could be called a place of custody. Equally, I have objected to the term *warehousing*, you see. Well, warehousing is an honorable profession in this country; you are willing to entrust the warehouse with your furniture because you know it will be properly kept and safe. No such conditions prevail in most of our large mass institutions.

Against this background then, spontaneous recognition of the rehabilitation potential of human beings evolved from World War II. The NIMH and all our rejuvenation of interest in mental health developed once it was learned that any man will break under sufficient pressure, but also that people who are utterly broken can be mended. I sometimes say, physically speaking, because many multiply handicapped veterans now have special drivers' licenses and with artificial limbs drive automobiles. Our physical rehabilitation program has been excellent as our mental rehabilitation programs moved forward at a very great rate.

Hidden Issues

Some of you have read about Polk State School and Hospital and the episode about difficult residents being caged. But there's another side of Polk. Polk is a main industry of its area. Polk is the largest employer in that area. And if you move Polk away, the grocery will close and the gas station will close and the whole economic picture of the area will change. People who have worked there for 20 or 25 years suddenly would be forced to move away. So when I speak of industry, we have a tremendous investment in this. The size of the investment I'd like to demonstrate to you by one example.

What broke the camel's back and led to the revolt in Pennsylvania that finally resulted in the first lawsuit of the right to education was the intention of the Department of Public Welfare to rehabilitate Pennhurst at a cost of $30 million but with the announced intention of scaling it down to an institution of 1000 people. Every one of the reconstituted beds would have cost the taxpayer $30,000; this in an institution that was already extant. Thirty thousand additional dollars into a rathole of an institution that once had a constituency in farm country and had lost it, and was now drawing employees from Philadelphia because that was the only source of employees for the daily care.

We are dealing with an industry that eats phenomenal amounts of tax dollars because the $30 million would not have come out of the general revenue but most likely out of special bond issues, a standard policy in most states. And before you have paid your bonds for $30,000 it has cost you $50,000 after interest charges. To stay for a moment with this picture, you could then take four of these people from Pennhurst and you would have $200,000 in tax money to build a house for them where they could live in the community. The per diem is steadily moving up now so that in New York very soon it will be $10,000 a year. If Pennsylvania will comply as it intends to with the standards of the Joint Commission for Accreditation it will soon also be at $10,000 a year. So not only would you spend $200,000 for these four people to have an abode for them but you would spend $40,000 to maintain them a year. Multiplied by hundreds of thousands of people gives you a fantastic amount of money.

In the mental illness field the figures are higher. At a point when I was involved in some investigation in Pennsylvania, Pennhurst had only a per diem of 7 dollars and some cents; a special small child phychiatry residential facility had a per diem of 70 dollars. The point I am making is that this establishment is one that affects large numbers of people and tremendous amounts of money. So what we are trying to do right now is to move away from this model. The difficulty we have in trying to move away from that model towards community care of the mentally disabled, in other words, the people who presumably are taken care of by the mental health programs, is our real problem.

In the process of this change, we are struggling for very little results. In Pennsylvania and Massachusetts, hundreds of thousands of dollars have remained unspent, because while the dollars are in the budget, we did not have either the people or the skills to really move into the community and do the things we are intending to do.

New Concepts in Mental Health

Normalization is a new concept that is badly misunderstood and invariably causes people to get needlessly excited. We have created conditions in the mental health field which distinctly deviated from the normal. In other words, we denormalized the life of human beings who are in these institutions. It is normal for people to do certain things in private. In the institution they are done in public. I remember that an institution in Connecticut had dormitories in a women's cottage they called a house that allowed anyone to simply look from the living room through a glass window right into the toilet area where, without partitions, there were 10 toilets. Usually, a person who would watch somebody sitting on the toilet is arrested. There are offenses against public morality. In the institution, we further such offenses. We make people live, sleep, and eat under conditions that are as denormalized as possible. When we speak of normalization, we want to move away from the denormalized conditions to conditions that are as normal as is appropriate for the particular person in question.

Deinstitutionalization is a process by which we are not just trying to take institutions and dump their contents onto a community; deinstitutionalization must be understood as our intention based on knowledge we have gained in recent years of avoiding the use of institutions. And, to me, much more crucial at the moment is to prevent the institutionalization of the person in the first place.

The problem of moving them out of the institutions is complicated by the fact that since we have created pathology in the institutions, we have some difficulty in deinstitutionalizing people. But for the moment it is much more important to prove that it is unnecessary to put people in institutions in the first place. The first community that has tried to do this in the field of mental retardation more vigorously than anybody has done in mental health is Omaha,

Nebraska. They want to take care of their people in their own community. To some extent, of course, the community mental health movement intended to do so, but it had difficulties, and as you know we still have our large state hospitals. We have gone fairly slowly.

You will hear about one other key word: *medical model*. The medical model needs to be written down in a particular way. The *medical* model runs fake hospitals, practices medicine that would be totally unacceptable in the general community, practices a psychiatry that is absolutely unknown in the community.

If a psychiatrist from a Philadelphia outpatient clinic, for example, were put in an institution for the mentally retarded where he would meet children, you might as well put him into China. He has no relationship to what goes on. His daily activities from 10:00 to 3:00 in the clinic in no way would relate to anything that would happen at that institution. In other words, the medical model in the institution is totally different

The medical model creates fake hospitals and fake patients. People are referred to as *patients*. They aren't sick; they don't run temperatures; their noses aren't stuffed up; their lungs are OK. They are ambulatory, but they are called patients. And just so you don't think I'm only being anecdotal, this is one of the real problems we have now, moving these people into the community. Fire laws are such that before you put these patients into this *community residence* you have to have a fire escape, a closed staircase (which in some houses just isn't possible), permanently lighted exit signs, and a sprinkler system. You could say to the fire marshall, "But please, the people being put in this house are people who will leave at 8:00 every morning with a lunchbox, go to some employment or some sheltered workshop, and come back later." And he says to you, "Buster, were they in the hospital? It says here they are patients." So you see, the medical model haunts us in the community now. We have created a ghost that is of great difficulty for us.

Being a *patient* is already a stigma of deviance, a labeling, a classification. I hope that somebody else can come and talk with you about some of these things. The labels one uses, for instance, applying to a retarded child the term "trainable," occurs because a school psychologist affixed a label to this child on the basis of an individual test possibly given in rather bad circumstances—probably the first time the child ever encountered such a person and possibly of emotional or physical health with other complicating circumstances. Suddenly this child is "trainable," which means we have a special program for him with which he is stuck. He never can get away because the other level we have, the most desirable level, educable, is not for trainables. So since you label him trainable, that's where he's going to be just as the nonambulatory child remains in the crib because he is nonambulatory. So since he's nonambulatory, nobody tries to get him to walk. And if you think I am exaggerating, then you may need to look at the system yourself, but that might make you a little sick.

These are fixed labels that were put on people with devastating results. I hope you read Rosenhan's article in *Science* (1973) about the group in the West who had committed themselves to a state hospital, and after they got there told the people that they were not sick, that they had tricked them; they said, "Pshaw. We know, we know. That's all right." And they were kept there and treated as sick people, no matter what they said. And they let them make the notes. They took records. Nobody stopped them. And they found out later on that this was in the clinical notes described as "writing behavior."

Another new conceptual framework has come up that deals with personal rights. You say, what's new about that? What's new about that is that mentally ill and retarded people were not endowed with rights. They officially had no rights. This was not just part of somebody's negligence, but they were not even considered persons. And, again, if you feel that I just make sort of loose conversation here, I could refer you to articles if you want to push me; only last fall I read an article which pointed out that people with an I.Q. below 20 were nonpersons. And so, if you thought that nonpersons were sort of a Communist political conception of people, we have some of the same kind of response in our own country, albeit sporadic and unsanctioned. The people I mentioned earlier who kept a woman seven years in confinement had learned institutional attitudes that allowed them to feel they were dealing with nonpersons. So there's a whole new concept of personal rights and legal rights; there are certain rights that one needs to have fulfilled right here and now; something more than just promissory notes against the future.

Using the Courts: A Contemporary Strategy

About three years ago an attorney from Philadelphia who was the chairman of the institutions committee of the (then) Pennsylvania Association for Retarded Children (PARC) came to me at Brandeis. I had over the years been many, many times here in Pennsylvania. I was a friend of the Association and helped them in many ways. They had come up by appointment for a day because they said, "We just don't know where next to turn." And they painted for me a little bit of the picture I mentioned to you, only more in detail.

For instance, they were aware of the exact location in Pennhurst where little children were being raped by older residents on a regular basis. There was a certain tunnel where this went on in the institution. Everybody knew it, and nothing was done about it. Protests had been made—just as the Association had made protests about the cages in Polk years ago—just as the Association had made protests before that until they finally closed the private institution where children were being maltreated, possibly to the point of being killed in the eastern part of the state. These all are matters of record. Still, children were being raped, and nobody did anything about it.

The Association knew that thousands of children were prevented from going to school. Children had a right to go to school. And they brought up any number of such things and said, "We are just at the end of the rope. We have gone to the Governor. We have gone to the Commissioner. We have protested. We have gone to the newspapers. We had the best of cooperation from television. They have done marvelous things in exposing, and nothing happens." And may I say here parenthetically that the one point where Bobby Kennedy totally failed was when he exposed the Willowbrook conditions. Three years before the thing finally came to a scandal, Bobby Kennedy had been in Willowbrook, and he made an expose, and went to the newspapers and television and nothing was done about it. It is this kind of rejection that the people at the Pennsylvania Association for Retarded Children—now the Pennsylvania Association for Retarded Citizens—had encountered.

My original training was in law. So I said to the people who came from PARC, "We have overlooked in the human services field one of the three branches of government, the executive, legislative, and the judicial. Courts are a helpful agency. Courts have a role to play in the human services field, and it's time we go to court." That was not simple. It is not easy to go in the court and make the Superintendent of Public Instruction a defendent; or to go in the court and sue Governor Rockefeller as we did in New York City; or to take the Secretary of Administration into court. The Association took a long time before they even gave us permission, which was finally granted. I hired an attorney who made an exhaustive study and came up with several possibilities. Interestingly, although he had the right-to-treatment suit at Pennhurst as well as other precedents, he chose the citizen's right to education, because the Association—whether they had learned from Bobby Kennedy's failure in New York or whether they instinctively felt it—wisely realized that the right to education was more readily something that the community could understand than the right of people in institutions not to be abused. Since institutional abuse is beyond the conception of the normal human being, it is simply denied.

The American Psychological Association, the American Psychiatric Association, the American Medical Association, the American Association of Social Workers never raised their voices, although they had innumerable members who knew about institutional abuse. Interestingly, the American Orthopsychiatric Association was the first to become an amicus curiae, that is, a friend of the court, in the *Rouse vs Cameron* case. In this case, Judge Basilon of the Federal Court of the District of Columbia found that a statutory right to treatment for mental patients in public hospitals did indeed exist.

We in Pennsylvania then also decided to go to court. We finally got the word. We went into the right-to-treatment suit. And this was the first event in the chain that led to the present state of affairs, where, right now, there are publications that keep us abreast every few months of the new legal activity in the field of mental health.

There was at the beginning a little story on each of the plaintiff's children, you see, who had been denied education. On the night before the Pennsylvania case was taken to court the attorney by long-distance checked the final text with me in Boston. And at my suggestion we made a change. The brief started out with these little vignettes, 5 lines ... Joe Dokes who has an I.Q. of 57, Mary Jones who has an I.Q. of 37, and so on. And I said, "Wait a minute. We are making a great mistake." And we said, "Joe Dokes who was assigned an I.Q. of 57." Some psychologist, right or wrong, maybe he was inexperienced, maybe he was a very experienced Ph.D.; on one certain day, under certain circumstances gave him, assigned to him an I.Q. That doesn't mean that he has it. This little change we made in the court case is a very significant one because it emphasizes the fact that the I.Q. score is a result of a process rather than an immutable trait of the child.

So, courts are part of our way of life. The greatest advantage we have in all of this was to confront the psychiatrists, physicians, psychologists, and social workers. The federal judiciary has two processes that are particularly fine: discovery and fact finding. After a complaint has been filed and the judge has assumed jurisdiction, you petition the other party through the court for documents, which you are entitled to see. That's the discovery process. That brings out the information and puts it on the table, you see. The judge later on decides what is significant, what is insignificant, and so on. But this is a very interesting thing.

Just to point out to you that we really entered into a new realm through using the discovery process with federal participation in the Willowbrook case the judge made an initial order and among other things ordered that immediately the recreation facilities be improved. You see, these people were locked up in these buildings. Willowbrook is on Staten Island in a beautiful natural setting and these people were never outside. The Department of Mental Hygiene came back some months ago, after a long interval, and said they had now complied with the new programs. The judge ordered 30 FBI agents into the institution who swooped down on the institution in one day. They found in this population of several thousand people 35 individuals outside the building on a sunny day. You see, I as a single expert witness can only go around building after building. They always can say, "Well, after you left they were out." But thirty FBI agents just made a finding that these people still were in prison, you see. By the way, in the Poplar case, the FBI agents went around and measured the temperature in that institution in Alabama where temperatures were almost unbearable for human beings. You see, it's up to me as a plaintiff to make sure that my facts are correct or the defendant will murder me. And so, out comes this fact-finding process and that is something the judiciary can do; the legislature could do it, but usually doesn't have time to do it. It is part of the judicial process.

The Right Not to Be Sterilized

Not every aspect of mental health is so easily adjudicated: take the whole area of birth control, sterilization, and abortion rights. Let me indicate to you how difficult it is with some hypothetical situations that have driven some of our law students up the wall. Down's syndrome is a chromosomal abnormality that now can be recognized in pregnancy. Down's syndrome can be recognized by taking some of the amniotic fluid and, tested by a very simple procedure. The first case I know of is the husband of a woman who is 40 and is pregnant and comes home and says, "Say, I talked in the office to some guys and they tell me that there's a real chance that at your age you can have a defective baby. And they have a new way of finding out about this, and I just wonder, Mary, whether—" And she says,

"Look Oscar, I know all about this. I know amniocentesis. I even can spell it, but there ain't no doctor putting a hole in my belly. Now just understand this." He says, "What do you mean. That's my child. I will have to bring it up." She says, "Nothing doing." He says, "I'll go into court." Well, of course he hasn't got a ghost of a chance with a court.

The second case is Susan who is more reasonable. She had amniocentesis, and the doctor calls her up and says, "Mrs. X, I have a little bit of disagreeable news for you. I just got the tests back and there's no question. The child you're carrying is a child with Down's syndrome. He will be born a defective baby."She says, "Oh, thanks a lot Doc. I'm glad to know. Thank you." He says, "Well, shall we set a date?" She says, "A date? What for?" He says, "For an abortion." She says, "Who's gonna have an abortion?" He says, "Mrs. X, you didn't understand me. Your child will be a child with Down's syndrome." She says, "Doctor, I understand it. My sister-in-law had one, and it was a surprise to her. It was a little difficult. But now I know and I'm very glad, and I can prepare myself, and I know things can be done for the baby. Thank you very much."

The doctor calls up the husband and says, "Look your wife has gone bananas. She wants to have this child." And he comes home and he says, "I'll go to court." She says, "Hah, you try." Has she got a ghost of a chance? So, in other words, this is a good situation to illustrate the difficulties of knowing what we should do about forcing people into situations.

The mentally retarded are relatively unlikely to have children. Furthermore, our evidence is that they not only don't procreate very readily, their heterosexual activities are on the whole very limited. The seriousness of the policy problem of sex among retardates is highly questionable, because as you know the law of nature moves, not towards the extreme, but toward the middle. It is not so that a woman who has an I.Q. of 70 is likely to have a child with an I.Q. of 60. Rather she has more likely chance to get an I.Q. of 80 or maybe 78 or whatnot, but she also may have normal offspring. And if you're sitting as a judge, by what right do you decide that she should be sterilized?

The odd feature of all this is that we are living in a different situation where sterilization is no longer essential. We have birth control methods which are adaptable to handicapped people. What is funny about this all to a man who has worked for forty years in this field is that we are arriving at this point of getting decisions against sterilization. These are decisions we need, but less urgently.

It has become fashionable to have a vasectomy. We have vastly more voluntary sterilization at this particular time than we ever had court-ordered ones. So maybe in a few years from now the whole idea of sterilization will be such that some of these people will make use of sterilization. I don't encourage mentally retarded individuals to have children, but it is not a major problem with me because I will try and deal with them in a realistic fashion. You're not just talking about procreation; you're talking about living together, managing a marriage, and so on. But basically the right to have sexual relations is not something you can remove from a person. We are coming in the criminal law to the whole issue of preventive detention, and so on, you see. You measure the value. You might prevent most offenses, and on the other hand, you might injure some people very severely. If you begin to make your decisions of ordering people not to have children, you're getting into a very dangerous field.

A Final Observation

In conclusion, may I point out to you that we have been very much prejudiced against the mentally retarded. Who has worried about the divorce rate in Hollywood and the havoc that it has played in the continual development of children in that situation? Are you ready to say because they lack the stability of marriage, Hollywood actors ought to be sterilized? In other words, what really are we afraid of in terms of the procreation? I think this is something we need to think of much more readily, but the main point is that we now give these people birth control methods, and we can in most states.

We sit down and talk with them and try to deal with this problem in realistic terms, and try to get from them an understanding of the situation, probe the problematics of bringing up children. And, at the moment, I feel this is a satisfactory way. We have, since about 1955, an ever-increasing number of mentally retarded in the community in sheltered workshops and other community situations. This has not been a major problem. The number of pregnancies, the number of children born to these people is, as we expected, rather limited. The real problem is with people who are *called* retarded, but who are really not retarded. They are school failures. They are people who have not had the advantage of education.

I said I will advise birth control. It's a very touchy problem in terms of permission and whether, when such people get pregnant, we will interfere with the pregnancy.

How would you feel? I am not going to ask you to vote, but suppose I would say to you, "How many of you would feel that amniocentesis should be reported to the State Department of Health, and the State Department of Health will decide whether to order an abortion?" How many of you would feel that this is desirable, that we should have state action? It's identifiable. How many of you would say that any woman coming for prenatal consultation to a doctor must have amniocentesis if she's over 40? It could be a state law. I think we are not quite ready for this yet.

THE COMMUNITY MENTAL HEALTH CENTER: A New Institutional Form for One Class of Social Problems

The federal government took the initiative in dealing with the extremes of institutionalization practices which the states had developed over the years. Federally based national studies of the costs and conditions of treatment and warehousing formed the bed on which the community mental health movement was conceived and delivered. Ira Goldenberg sees the basis of federal responsibility in the competitive structure of our society. The win-lose essence of the distribution of goods and power of neccessity produces social casualties. The fact that a certain percentage of the population will be unemployed is one dimension of the competitive process. Given this, society has an obligation to those who have been injured by playing according to the rules, and even to those who have engaged in criminal acts, which had as their ends the gaining of values offered as incentives to engage in the struggle.

Robert Reiff is credited with being the catalytic agent of the Swampscott Conference which sought means to implement the idea of community mental health that federal legislation used to deal with the dilemmas caused by institutional care. One procedure is to prevent institutionalization and the other to provide the means for deinstitutionalization. The latter was to be based on psychotropic drugs and community based half-way houses. The former was to be based on broad ranging attacks on the social structure, attacks which attempted to produce social change conducive to the mental health of problem ridden publics. These two tacks formed the basis of the community mental health movement.

Leonard Hassol is a successful strategist for effective changes of the community structure. Yet, it is his remarks that lead to a fundamental critique of community mental health as the staging area of community change efforts. Among other searching questions are, do a lot of little victories add up to social change or simply to patching up and preserving the already existing community structure? Further, even if the community structure were altered and augmented, how much of the social costs can we rightly ask the community to bear? For the fact still remains that it is the dynamics of a national economy and not strictly local factors which form the basis of many emotional problems and, therefore, the federal and state governments still have a share of the responsibility.

Let us suppose with the speaker that our society is founded on three assumptions about goods and power. The first assumption is that the absolute amount of goods and power is finite at any given point in time. The second is that under no conditions will the goods and power be equally distributed in the population. The third is the assumption that the sense of self-worth of an individual is determined by his or her ability to acquire and hold goods and power.

Suppose also that the formal social institutions of education, mental health, law, social welfare, and employment consistently discriminate in their process of legitimatizing those who may acquire goods and power. The question becomes, what is the role of mental health services in such a society? Dr. Ira Goldenberg outlines and critiques four traditional responses: The system as consolator, as elector of tokens, as healer of systemoclasts, and as messiah of missing persons. Perhaps the mental health system presents concrete images of our historical stage of evolution which conscience and morality will push us beyond.

Chapter 7

ON THE CREATION OF THE NEW SOCIAL SETTINGS

Ira Goldenberg

In the Shadow of the 1960s

Most of us involved in the areas of change today are acting, willingly or unwillingly, under the cloud of emotions that were generated in the 1960s, and that we have not been able to resolve. Let me be more specific. I think most of us, whether we know it or not, are dealing with two fairly powerful human emotions that are influencing the way in which we think about problems and the ways in which we conceive of trying to solve them. Those emotions are fear and depression, and I think they come out of experiences of the 1960s that we have not been able to resolve.

In the 1960s, America was at a point when the reexamination of itself was no longer considered an act of treason, but rather a sacred right. And we had two things going for us in the 1960s; we created the image of a new kind of leadership that in one way or another was more committed to study what it was that was paining America. Second, we were confronted with the specter of potential programs that were essentially going to deal with what most people considered to be the elitist, racist, sexist nature of modern society. The fascinating thing about that period was that, instead of either of those two things materializing into any substantive programs, we became aware of two things. The first was the incredible violence that lies at the heart of the American experience. I think white, middle-class, alienated, and liberal America became aware of the violence. The assassinations of John Kennedy, Malcolm X, Martin Luther King, and Robert Kennedy finally brought home to all the young activists the fact that not only did violence exist, but that individuals could be summarily executed in ways that were both public and in ways that could be personalized. We came out of the 1960s with the first realization by a group of people who hadn't realized it before, directly, that this was indeed an incredibly violent culture. That violence has carried over into the 1970s into a kind of quiet, muted, ongoing fear.

The second experience of the 1960s that I think we're still trying to come to grips with today is the feeling of being impotent. The programs of the 1960s promised, in glowing rhetoric, a great number of things, and whether that rhetoric was honest or not, the promise was public. The War on Poverty was going to do away with the victims and the institutional sources of individual victimization. And what were the results of these massive programs and so-called human and institutional renewal? Nothing. They didn't change a thing. Poverty was not done away with. Poverty wasn't even approached seriously.

Now when you put those two things together, you essentially form a context for attempts to change things which will be called more mature, more responsible, and less conflict producing, but whose outcomes have nothing to do with being more mature, more responsible, or more skilled. For a brief period of time, America was at the point of almost being able to transcend its historical consciousness. Instead of doing so, it recoiled from that moment and, almost as if guided by reflex, it destroyed the symbols of approaching liberation and essentially put the stamp of futility on the process of liberation. Violence and impotence are two very disturbing emotions to deal with, especially for those of us who have tried to stay in the mental health field. Given that as the background, what I'd like to talk about is how one begins to think about change— whether change means changing existing institutions or creating alternatives in terms of the American experience. For me, this involves trying to conceptualize clearly for myself—in ways that go beyond rhetoric—what America really is. What are the forces I'm trying to understand? What are the forces I'm trying to change? What are the conditions that confront me when I think about the American experience? I'd like to try to describe that a bit and then try to suggest some of the implications of this particular conceptual analysis for what people actually do.

Goods and Power

There are certain historical values that characterize the American society: and which then get translated into characterizing the American experience. Whether or not I agree with those values is not the issue here. Alright, I'm not saying this is America as it should be. I'm saying this is America as I've experienced it to be. Now I think we live in a country which by and large is dominated by two themes that have not changed over the last 200 years. Those themes are that the most important things in life are goods and power. Let me try to represent this state of affairs graphically as a figure in the shape of an hourglass. Now, in the upper compartment of the glass are the values of goods and power. Goods means those material, transferable, exchangeable commodities which, if possessed in sufficient number, enable one to deal with the question of survival as well as the question of meaning. For example, if I'm always having to try to get two bucks for food to make it through the day, I have very little energy or time left to think about "the bigger questions or the meaning of my life." But goods are simply those material things that in one way or another determine how comfortably an individual lives. That could be money or something else. Power is the ability to control one's own destiny and/or to have dominion over others, so that one's efforts to insure one's own survival become minimal. Power is the ability to control the conditions under which one's existence takes place.

Theoretical Assumptions of American Society

American society has made three particular assumptions about goods and power. The first assumption is that the overall, the absolute, amount of goods and power that is available in the society in any particular point in time, is finite. In other words, the assumption in our society is that goods and power are exhaustible, and that they are not self-generating. The second assumption is that under no conditions will the existing amount of goods and power be shared among all citizens; this is a very critical assumption. The third assumption is that the reference point for the analysis of how goods and power are acquired, used, or misused is the individual. America is predicated on the assumption that the individual determines his own value (or lack of it) as a human being, in terms of his ability to acquire and hold goods and power.

Now the fascinating thing about these values and the assumptions that lie below these values is that they invariably set up what has been called an exploitative and competitive society. I'm not talking now about capitalism versus some other form of economic system; I'm talking in purely conceptual terms. When you make the assumption of scarcity, nonsharability, and individual effort, a system that has to be exploitative and competive is set up: where one person's acquiring depends on another person's losing. So it is a competitive society in that everyone competes for a limited amount of nonsharable goods, but it's also an exploitative society which says that in order to get more, one has to eventually get it at the expense of someone else.

Down in the lower compartment of our hourglass are the people. The most democratic thing about our society, the true meaning of the term democracy in our society, is that everyone in our society from the moment of birth, regardless of race, creed, color, religion, or country of national origin gets the same message that goods and power are the most important things in life. Even if they don't internalize the basic assumption—they get the clear message that is transmitted by the media, i.e., any of the pathways and paths by which and through which the message is communicated to people. This is not only through television, but through legend, story, the written word, the cultural artifact, or any other means. What comes through to people is the message from the moment of birth that your value as an individual will ultimately be determined in practical terms by how much goods and power you have been able to acquire through your life. That is democracy; everyone gets the message equally.

It is interesting, for example, to note that in most social welfare programs in the allocation of welfare in the city, welfare recipients are encouraged to buy televisions. And, in some places, that becomes the way in which social workers begin to interact with people—the question of helping them get the right television. The powerful message of the core values of the society is communicated equally to everyone from the earliest point on. What is also communicated is assumption that all people are going to start their pursuit of goods and power from a position of equity. What is communicated to people is that everyone is going to start out from a common position of a relative lack of goods and power. That is not true, of course; and, recently, that's not even been attempted to be communicated to people. But the initial assumption is that this goods-and-power message comes down to people, all of whom are going to start their trek up the hourglass towards the goods and power from the same point, so that whether you're rich or poor, white or black, male or female, everybody gets the same message and presumably is inspired to start striving toward the same goal.

Inequity of Access

In an exploitative, competitive society everyone does not start at the same point on the starting line. Whether you want to talk about it in the 'simplest terms—through inheritance—or through much more sociologically complex terms—that certain individual groups are singled out and become more exploited over time than other groups—this is what the reality is. Of course, this historical reality does not come down to people who are "all at the same starting point." You know, if you're rich, white, and male, you're probably a lot closer to what can be considered the access channel, the neck of the hourglass, towards the goods and power than if you're poor, nonwhite, and nonmale. Now that is not only a result of historical accident, it is also the result of pernicious intent. Slavery, the importation of black people, for example, was an economic move, the result of which was to create an encapsulated population which, in point of fact, over the years, has been kept encapsulated.

I am not really interested in which group is the most exploited, women, blacks, or poor whites. Rationales can be developed for a sexist, racist, or class analysis of group exploitation, all of which are equally valid. All that's important to me is that, both through historical accident and pernicious intent, certain whole parts of the population are rendered inoperative—long before the message of what they were to be striving for reaches them. It is not true that a poor white has the same opportunity as a rich white. Historical accident and pernicious intent make that impossible.

The Function of Existing Institutions

Everyone gets and believes the same message and then starts the striving upward. A society based on the assumptions and treasuring the values I described cannot really afford to have a totally open society. It doesn't follow from the consequences of the assumptions. So, what we have in our society is the formal social institution. Those formal social institutions—and there are many of them—include the educational, mental health, legal, social welfare, and employment systems. The job of the formal social institution is willingly or unwillingly, to monitor the progression of people in their striving upward.

The function of the formal social institutions in our society—as in any society—is to play a legitimizing and socializing role in terms of determining who it is that starts from this position of presumed powerlessness and makes it up through the access channel to where the goodies are. Now the important thing to note is that if the society is dominated by certain values, assumptions and their ensuing behaviors, then the formal social institutions must mirror those very assumptions and behaviors and must project them.

It should come as no surprise (nor should it be allowed to fit into anyone's conception of the world in paranoid terms) for me to say that if the society and its institutions, because of historical accidents and pernicious intent, does in fact turn out to be racist, sexist, and elitist, it is not because the legitimizing or socializing functions that the social institutions perform must be consistent with the underlying ethos of the system as a whole. Thus it's fascinating to note that in every one of the five critical socializing and legitimizing social institutions mentioned above, the same groups are oppressed in the same way. For example, we know that the administration of justice is inconsistent and too often has little to do with justice. I can give you the data that show that poor people get longer sentences than rich people. We know that white-collar criminals are treated differently from blue-collar criminals. We know, for example, that in law, the poor, the nonwhite get the worst treatment. We know that the psychotherapeutic practices in the mental health professions, however questionable in total, are least effective with those who are uneducated or less educated, who are poor, and who are black. We know that the school system, tracks poor whites, blacks, and females out of that track which leads to the universities, which supposedly lead to the ability to acquire greater goods and power.

We know that the social welfare system systematically destroys those that it is supposed to help by teaching people that they are dependent and powerless. We know for a fact that if employment is a problem nationwide, it is a catastrophe for poor whites, nonwhites, and females.

The fascinating thing to see is that it's not just one institution: if it were just one institution that was systematically discriminating against a particular class of people, one could say that was to be expected on the basis of chance, but the fact that the same pattern holds true in all of the formal social institutions. It cannot be an accident. That's not to say it has to do with conscious malicious intent on the part of the individuals. What it *does* have to do with is the fact that those social institutions mirror in their own socializing and legitimizing functions the values of the society as a whole. So, if the society is racist, sexist, and elitist, all of the social institutions have to be.

The Role of Mental Health Systems

Consolator

Now let me show you how I think this happens in that part of the social institutions that I know the best, the mental health systems. What happens to that individual when, as is most often the case, he or she realizes that the competition is sick, that the society is not as open as its rhetoric would like us to believe? How does that relate to how the mental health professions function? That's what I want to kind of try and characterize. The individual finally realizes that— hey, I am never going to get through that access channel. I'm never really going to get a part of the goodies that I've been taught to want and taught to associate my self-worth with. What happens to that individual?

One option is that the individual adjusts to a position of relative powerlessness. One possibility and probably the predominant behavioral option chosen is to realize that they won't make it. The function of mental health professionals is to help people adjust to conditions they have no control over.

So first of all, there is the notion that most mental health services that have been made available to people who are in this position, have been services geared toward helping individuals adjust to external conditions and have not been geared toward mobilizing individuals to change those external conditions.

Elector of Tokens

The second function of the mental health profession is seeking out, encouraging, and supporting token or representative achievers. Let me be a little more specific about this second option. I am convinced that a system which is basically closed, but purports to be open, needs its tokens. In order to maintain the myth of its openness, the mental health professions have functioned to seek out, help, encourage, and support numbers of people from disadvantaged groups to make it. Mental Health, therefore, helps selected individuals make it through the system.

Let me give you an example. When I went to school in New York, I was terrible, probably one of the worst kids in the public school system. My parents didn't speak English, and we were always on welfare. They were afraid of the school, and I very rarely went to school, partly because I hated it, and partly because I had more fun not going. My mother would get called into school twice a semester, and each time she would be told in English, which she couldn't understand and, therefore, it impressed her even more, that I was one of two things: either mentally retarded or pathologically disturbed. And that's what she finally got; she would bring neighbors to interpret for her. My mother was always angry, by the way, when she was called to school because it meant, if she was working, she would be giving up a day's work. That's a lot to give up when you're not working all that often. So I remember that my mother was told the best thing that you can try to do with this wretched thing that somehow came out of you is either try to get him into some kind of help, some institution somewhere, or, if we can at least keep him in school without killing him or allowing him to kill someone else, we'll try to get him into machine and metal trades high school, which was where the dummies were sent to learn a vocation.

Now, a fascinating thing happened around 1944 when the I.Q. extravaganza occurred in this country. As it turned out, I happened to be in school that day. Many of my friends, by the way, whom I consider to this day to be much brighter than I ever was, were not in school that day. I somehow took this test and in a period of about two weeks my whole life changed. I still don't know what the test said, you know, but all of a sudden, my mother was called to school and no longer told that I was either crazy or mentally retarded. She was told that I wasn't being challenged. All of a sudden, the crazy dumb kid becomes the unchallenged smart kid. I couldn't read any better nor could I write any better. I was still getting into fights, but, now, all of a sudden, I was the recipient of more services than you could believe. I had tutors. I remember once when opening the door when I was about to take off and not go to school, that my teacher was standing outside my door and took me by the hand and walked me to school for three straight weeks. I had social workers in the family. I had educational tutors in the school. I was the recipient of more compensatory education service in the next year of my life than I think any kid was in the 1960s who got into a compensatory education program.

The fact was that my whole life changed. I'm quite sure to this day that I wouldn't have gotten through school, and I wouldn't have gotten anywhere without that test. It was not something that would have happened anyway. I consider that to have been an accident that I was fortunate enough to have been the beneficiary of. But the fact that it was done that way makes me feel all the more strongly that it was important for the social system we live with to have a significant number of people from groups that would traditionally be excluded from the social hierarchy helped into that hierarchy to provide additional legitimacy for that hierarchy in the last analysis. I maintain that there were kids brighter than me who didn't take that test, and I think the fact that I was lucky, rather than invalidating what I'm trying to say, highlights it.

I am not saying that a small group of people decide what's going to happen to everybody. What I *am* saying is that it is systematically important in this society that we see significant representation at relatively low levels, of the goods and power hierarchy. It is important to have significant numbers of disadvantaged people make it somewhat through the system in order to add legitimacy to the system itself. So that search and support of tokens in large numbers has been a very important part of mental health professions.

Healer of Systemoclasts

A third function involves the person who is not going to make it through and who chooses the option to try to break out of the ordinary competitive system. We generally call that criminal behavior, because if you're not going to make it up the ladder, another option is to try to break out—to try to acquire goods and power illegitimately where they have been denied legitimately. One can take a look at all forms of criminal behavior, especially blue-collar criminal behavior, as the attempt to acquire the very same goods and power that one has been denied through the access channels that are legitimizing society.

Some people go so far as to view a lot of criminal behavior as revolutionary, that is, as a protest against "the system." That may or may not be the case. The fact of the matter is, in many instances, what is called criminal behavior is the attempt to acquire the goods and power that have been denied via the "legitimate" process. What has been the response in the mental health profession towards that option? We have played, and we are continuing to play, an increasingly greater role in diagnosing, labeling, separating, and treating the offender. One of the biggest new pushes in the area of the mental health professions is our involvement with the criminal justice system. I'm not talking just about in prisons. Very few judges now make decisions without the help of some kind of clinical intervention; We don't want to punish; we want to "treat", which somehow seems more humane than punishment. The fact of the matter is that our function for those who try to break out of the system is to isolate, label, diagnose, and treat.

Some forms of treatment now are becoming frightening. The growth of behavior modification, in ways that haven't examined some of the crucial underlying political and moral issues, is potentially dangerous. The growth of psychotechnology is going to be, I think, one of the key issues in the next 10 to 15 years in this society. The use and the application of behavioral science data—research on the development of conformance behavior is not going to be in the hands of the police; it's going to be in the hands of the behavioral scientists or the mental health professional. I've spent a lot of time in the last three years working with people in the criminal justice system, and I am frankly very frightened about a great deal of what I see being done by, for, and with mental health professionals.

None of the three approaches I have outlined has anything to do with changing the system. They all have to do either with changing the individual or somehow helping the individual cope with the system over which he has no control.

As Messiah of Missing Persons

There is one final function. The person who isn't going to get anywhere and is either too scared or too wise to try to break out illegally often falls through the grate; he can choose to disappear into drugs and alcohol. It's been interesting to note that there's a difference between the drugs consumed by poor people as opposed to the drugs consumed by rich people. Poor people have traditionally been on "hard stuff" because it "turns off" the environment. Up until recently, alienated white middle-class kids who have been getting on drugs, have been using drugs that intensify the environment, So, some people will fall through and will become what I call involuntarily alienated, distinguishing them from those who want to "turn off" the environment and are voluntarily alienated.

What has been the response of the mental health professions to those who fall into drug addiction and alcoholism as a way of trying to survive what has become an optionless existence? The traditional response in the mental health professions has been to save these people. My profession has, in many cases, played the "savior." Grab this person before he falls through the grate and save him even if he has fallen through the grate. Saved for what? That's not a question that concerns most of us. But save him. This is the fourth traditional response of the mental health profession.

Some Conclusions

If I have this kind of an overall conception of the American experience, what does this mean to me in terms of being a change agent, or in terms of getting involved in the development of services or the creation of alternatives? Well, what it means is that I can no longer do any one of those four things. I can no longer support tokens, adjust people to mediocrity, save people from their alienation, or label and treat people for their criminality. Maybe my role in terms of where I am in the system ought to be confined much more toward trying to make the mental health professionals aware of how they have been playing their role in ways that work against effective change. A very good description of that role appears in William Ryan's book *Blaming the Victim* (1971), a masterful book which literally and very persuasively tells exactly how the behavioral scientist has created and indeed carried out the theories and the programs which continually blame the victim for his own victimization. That's an important kind of consciousness-raising book, not for the victim, but for the helpers. Well, what Bill Ryan is doing is trying to effect change in his own profession.

A second option is to try to change the width or narrowness of the access channel to goods and power. One of the things that mental health professionals can do is to arbitrarily begin legitimizing people they wouldn't legitimize in the past. For no other reason other than to do it! And why not? That brings with it a long-term perspective on change and has to do with things like what happens when you flood the system with people who would not normally get through?

A third possibility, of course, is to attack directly the underlying values and assumptions of the system itself, which makes creation of alternatives very important. Most alternatives that are created, in one way or another, have to be predicated on a reanalysis of the particular values that underlie the system. Are we creating new towns, for example, essentially, to perpetuate a value system that we have no control over, or do we create new towns differently in an attempt to develop alternative values which are as appropriate for poor people as they seem to be for rich people? Rich people are the people interested in examination of values because they have the luxury of time to do it. Maybe new towns ought to take very seriously the notion of the alternative conceptual basis for a new town, and not after the town is built, but before the town is built. It would lead to great differences in who gets involved in the building process, with that kind of power, and with what kinds of resources. There is a great deal more to be said, but let me conclude by saying that I have been making an in-process kind of analysis. What I hope it does is to make a little clearer what, to my mind, has been the American experience and the options it gives rise to in terms of what mental health people ought to do. The options are not all given by the analysis. No analysis invariably brings with it all the options; but I've tried to outline a few of the most important ones.

Robert Reiff, instigator, goad, and critic of community psychology, argues that distributive justice and rationality are the two values on which to base movements for the changes in the social structure necessary to raise the quality of individual and community life. In recounting the growth of the community mental health movement and the adoption of systems thinking by psychologists who would work at the community level, Reiff counsels caution in defining primary prevention as a goal, chides psychologists and sociologists alike for being blinded by "scientific isomorphism," and asserts the need for a new breed of professionals who would be the change agents of tomorrow.

Chapter 8

RECENT TRENDS AND PROSPECTIVE PROBLEMS IN COMMUNITY MENTAL HEALTH

Robert Reiff

Origins of Community Mental Health Theory

One of the interesting roots of the idea of community mental health grew out of a U.S. Army study in which it was demonstrated that if a soldier experienced a breakdown on the front lines and was sent to the rear to a convalescent home or a hospital he would more likely take months to recover or might never recover. But if he was kept on the front line and given some emergency treatment or a few days' rest and then was sent back to the front, he would recover more quickly. That was one of the origins of the idea of getting the mentally ill back into the community and functioning as quickly as possible.

Another reason for the thrust toward community mental health was the changing attitude of society toward mental illness, and the idea that mental illness was something to be hidden. Traditionally, state mental hospitals were situated 20 miles outside the city boundary, where they were well concealed. This tended to reinforce the concept of mental illness as a stigma. People were ready to accept the idea that mental illness was just another illness and that the mentally ill can learn to function while continuing to live in the community.

The contribution of England to psychiatry where social and community emphasis have become very popular, has also had an important influence on American attitudes. But because of the differences in psychiatric ideology between the two countries, the English concept underwent a significant change in America. In the United States, psychiatry is based firmly on a Freudian orientation. There are a large number of psychiatrists who may not be Freudians, however, but, in general, almost all the schools in the United States have a Freudian orientation.

In England there is a strong genetic approach. Many people in England feel that an illness such as schizophrenia is genetic and cannot be cured. Consequently, it is treated like any other permanent injury. The concept of rehabilitation of the mentally ill in England is similar to the concept of rehabilitation of the paraplegic in this country. As in physical rehabilitation, the idea is to get the handicapped person functioning as quickly as possible and to the best of his ability. In community mental health, the idea is to get the mentally ill functioning and back in the community as quickly as possible, i.e., restoring them to some kind of functional level.

The basic philosophy of the community mental health movement is rehabilitative. And, while we don't have the same theoretical bias as the English, we still treat the mentally ill in America like paraplegics, giving up the idea of treatment as "cure" and organizing treatment services as rehabilitation.

The Evolution of Community Programs

It is necessary to make a distinction between community and social psychiatry as a theory, and community mental health as a program in this country. It is an important distinction. I have been talking about the theoretical basis for community mental health which rests on social and community psychiatry theory. While related theoretically, the community mental health program in this country had ambiguous goals from the very beginning. This ambiguity has created many difficulties for the community mental health movement in this country.

Primary Prevention

Historically, whenever there has been a shift in the mental health movement in this country, it has always been accompanied by a cry for the need for a greater emphasis on primary prevention. Nearly a century ago when the Mental Hygiene Association became the Mental Health Association, one of its major declarations was that what was needed was an association which emphasized primary prevention. When the community mental health movement was launched, there was again a great deal of verbal emphasis on primary prevention. But like all primary prevention movements of the past, it has simply slipped away. There's little that can be called primary prevention in the community mental health movement today, and, in fact, it never has been mounted successfully in this country. I believe that primary prevention is a contradiction in terms and is not possible given our present Freudian-based orientation in mental health.

Throughout history, there's been a great deal of lip service paid to primary prevention, but it's never been implemented. The result has been an ambiguity about the major objectives and goals of the community mental health movement in the United States. If the goal is primary prevention, then the target group is the entire population of society and the objective is to prevent the development of mental illness.

Tandem Targets: The Poor and the Hospitalizable

Primary prevention, it seems to me, directs itself toward the prevention of an illness before the illness exists, which means that it's directed toward those who are not ill, not the casualties of society, but to all those in society who are at risk of developing a mental illness. When the community mental health programs were planned and were developing their programmatic styles, there were some community mental health centers who took the position that the target group were those who were in greatest risk of developing a mental illness, the poor, the low-income groups, etc. There were a number of community mental health centers, on the other hand, who defined their target group as those who were in the greatest risk of hospitalization. This means, in most cases, those who already had the beginnings of a mental illness, but the major objective was, nevertheless, to keep them out of the hospital.

These were two very important directions in the beginning of the community mental health movement: one in which a good deal of attention was given to trying to keep people out of the hospital. Coincident with the development of the community mental health movement was the development of the poverty movement under the Office of Economic Opportunity. The Office of Economic Opportunity gave a great deal of support to the view which held that the poor were its primary target. They supported a number of community mental health center programs from antipoverty funds.

Just to give you a sense of this ambivalent situation, the Albert Einstein College of Medicine had two community mental health centers: one held that the poor were its primary target and worked toward developing programs for the poor, and another which held that the primary target was those in the greatest risk of hospitalization. In the same institution we had this dichotomy that resulted in very different programs. For example, nonprofessionals recruited from the poor were used extensively in one program, while the other employed no nonprofessionals.

What happened historically was that many of those who were interested in the poor as a primary target had a great deal of political, staff, and community difficulty. There were many explosions and crises. As a result of the political risks of working with the poor in order to improve the quality of life, there is now a reaction in which almost all community mental health programs have given up their preventive objectives and are now oriented toward those in greatest risk of hospitalization. This is an issue that will have to be faced in the future. The outcome will depend on what funds are available for an orientation towards considering the poor as the primary target, as well as the degree to which the mental health professionals are politically naive, a factor which was one of the major causes of the explosions in those community mental health centers that wanted to engage in social change for the poor.

Parallel Developments in Community Psychology

Concomitant with this development in the community mental health movement, there was the development of the community psychology movement within psychology. In 1965, about 35 psychologists got together at Swampscott, Massachusetts, to try to figure out what important things psychologists should do in the renewed community mental health movement. (Bennett, et al., 1966). There, everybody seemed to have the same idea at once; it was one of the few conferences that I ever attended that I thought was worthwhile, and where I experienced some professional growth. It was a time when a number of people were becoming disenchanted with the one-to-one relationship in therapy. They were becoming uncomfortable about the neglect by psychology of the poor and the needy in society. They were also becoming unhappy in their professional role as therapists with the kind of success they were achieving in that role.

And so we came together at Swampscott and we all felt much the same way: we had to develop a new orientation in psychology, not to replace clinical psychology, but as a new thrust of psychology. That new development, as we saw it then, consisted of a turning away from the one-to-one relationship of therapy to what was called the systems approach. There has probably been more confusion about the concept of the systems approach than almost any other concept in the whole area of mental health today. The systems approach was supposed to be the answer to the disenchantment with the one-to-one relationship, and it was also supposed to be the answer to the social role of the psychologist as a change agent.

There was a heavy interest in developing the role of the psychologist as a change agent, and the impossibility of doing this on a one-to-one basis was obvious to everybody. Systems were defined as anything from a family to a group, to an organization, to the whole of society: any group of more than three people was defined as a system.

Another idea ensuing from the Swampscott Conference was the concept of action. We felt that psychologists for too long had confined themselves to observe rather than participate in the programs that were being designed for social change. Out of this feeling the concept of the participant-conceptualizer was promulgated. A psychologist should participate in action programs while at the same time conceptualizing what he was doing.

That was the thrust of the Swampscott Conference. What has happened since is an interesting lesson in institutional change. Many, perhaps a majority, of the people who adopted community psychology as a desirable approach came from clinical psychology. Many of them then began to work in the community mental health centers. As a result, community psychology began to take on the appearance of a specialty of clinical psychology, i.e., a community approach to clinical psychology. Many clinical psychologists joined the American Psychological Association's Division of Community Psychology. Being a member of the Division of Community Psychology implied that one was competent to work in a community mental health center, and that's where all the jobs were. Consequently, the Division of Community Psychology became a job opportunities movement for psychologists. The Division of Community Psychology is still plagued with that problem. There has never been any real conceptual clarity about what community psychology is, where community psychology is going, where it ought to go, and how it differs from clinical psychology. I was one of the founders of the division of community psychology and its first president. That problem has been plaguing me ever since the division was organized.

Toward a System Perspective

I have tried to develop a conceptual framework which helps to clarify where we are in the field of community mental health and where I think we ought to go. In the beginning of community psychology and community mental health, we talked about working with systems. Even today, if you go to any community mental health center and ask them what they are doing that's different from an ordinary psychiatric clinic, they would say they work with systems rather than with individuals. And if you ask, "What do you do with systems that is different from what you do with individuals?" "Well, we do group work; we offer consultation—there are any number of techniques which we use in order to help individuals." "You mean if you work with a group and you're helping individuals, then you're working with a system?" "Yes, we're working with a system." So this confusion goes on and on all the way through much of the thinking of psychologists in community mental health. I want to describe a design that I think helps to clarify this issue.

Operational Levels

Any society is organized on several different levels. From the viewpoint of mental health professionals, let us call them *operational* levels. They represent the areas in which a professional can operate to effect change. There's the individual level, the one-to-one relationship. Then there is the group or family level, above the group or family is the organization level, and above the organization is the institution level.

I have to explain what I mean by "institution" here. Institution in our language is used in two different ways. We speak of the college as an institution; we speak of many formal organizations as institutions; and then we speak of institution in the other sense when we speak of the institution of the family or the institution of law. That's a different use of the term institution. Here I'm using institution as a higher level of organization, meaning an organization of organizations.

For example, under organization I would include a public school. Under institution I would include the public school *system*. Then there is, of course, the community level, and the society level.

The mistake that many of the people in community mental health are making is to say, "We're not going to work with the individual anymore. We're going to work with communities. Therefore, we are working with systems." But when it comes down to what they are doing with systems, we find out they're doing the same thing no matter what level they're working at.

Behavior-shaping Factors

Here I have to explain something further for you. Human behavior seems to be shaped by number of factors. One is the disposition of a person, that is, his intrapsychic and intrapersonal condition, those dispositional factors which make up "the person." Another factor which shapes his behavior is his immediate milieu or situation. You behave in a lecture room in a certain way, because the situation requires you to behave that way. These situational factors shape one's behavior. Social structures also shape human behavior, for example, the institution of the family.

When a married couple has difficulties and they agree to separate or get a divorce, these difficulties may be due entirely to dispositional factors or with the immediate milieu; but they may also have something to do with the social structure. When 50 percent of the marriages begin to dissolve in separation and divorce, one can suspect legitimately that the social structure has a lot more to do with the divorce than dispositional or situational factors.

Dynamics of the System: Effecting Change

If one were to lay out a grid with the different levels of social organization mentioned previously along one dimension and these behavior-shaping factors along the other, something very interesting turns up. Let's say you're working with a group or a family in a community mental health center. Where is it—at what operational level—that you're trying to effect change? One can operate on the level of a system, but that doesn't mean that one is then producing system change. This is the fallacy of most of the mental health professionals who think that if they operate on a particular level, then they are automatically producing change at that level. That is not true. It helps to clarify that issue. You can operate on a community level but still be interested in producing changes in the dispositional factors of an individual. Simply because you are working with systems does not necessarily mean that you are producing system change. Most of the people in community mental health are operating at different system levels but are interested primarily in producing individual change.

What does the community work that is being done by community mental health centers consist of? Usually it means putting a psychiatrist or a psychologist in the public school system to look for early signs of mental illness and then treating the child individually. It's secondary prevention in most cases: early case finding, outreach, etc., with the primary aim of early treatment of those individuals who are going to be ill or who already have been. The characteristic with which professionals justify calling this activity community work is that they operate at the community level.

Of course, in order to accomplish situational or social structural change, one may decide that before anything can be accomplished, some kind of relationship with some individuals must be established. That's merely a tactic. I don't think it's a necessary stage that you have to go through every time you want to accomplish change in the situation or in the social structure. It would depend on what the problem is and what the situation is. But I would not propose that everybody has to be a clinician. I would say, as a matter of fact, that if you are a clinician, with a primary emphasis on the intrapsychic and intrapersonal definition of problems, that it is an obstacle to defining the problem in a way that enables you to act in either of these two other areas. So I would not propose that we all become clinicians.

One of the institutional laws in our society is that people tend to define problems in terms of their own skills. If you're a clinician diagnosing an organizational problem it is most likely to be diagnosed as a problem in interpersonal relations or something having to do with somebody who's a little emotionally disturbed. If you're a clinician in the community, then the problem is almost always defined in terms of either intrapsychic or intrapersonal variables. And this really makes a difference on how you operate and whether you're able to accomplish situational or social structure change.

If you're constantly defining problems in terms of intrapersonal and intrapsychic conditions, then your solution will tend to be individual or dispositional change. How do you deal with a problem of people defining problems in terms of their own professional skills? I would say that the wider repertoire of skills you have at your disposal, the less chance there is of your doing that.

Let us consider then, an example of how a change in social structure could occur without any dispositional change. Much depends, of course, on what one calls dispositional change. If, for example, someone says that people, as a result of the energy crisis, are becoming depressed or angry, and that is a dispositional change, then of course the answer is that there is no change in the social structure which doesn't produce a dispositional change. But a person may react with more anger at one time or less anger at another time, but that doesn't change his psychodynamic structure. I am defining dispositional factors here in the more general sense, that is, in terms of the psychodynamic structure of the person rather than in the more common usage of the word meaning mood or temper.

Let me say that it seems to me that the primary goal of most social change agents would be in the social structure and the intermediate goals would be situational. In other words, it's very difficult to change social structures completely from the top. One would have to begin to operate in the immediate milieu. This is the area that I would like to see community psychologists begin to work in. This raises a whole series of questions about whether the clinician is able to work in this area, because if it is true, as the prevailing theory holds, that mental illness in our society is etiologically related to the social structure or to social conditions, then, it seems to me, primary prevention is a matter of social reform. Social reform is something which clinicians know absolutely nothing about, and, therefore, they should not be playing games with it.

Social workers tend to look at these problems in a different way than psychologists and psychiatrists. This used to be the primary orientation of social workers, but when the prestige and the popularity of therapy became something to be sought after, then social workers abandoned that whole orientation and became therapists indistinguishable from psychologists. There is a movement today to move social work back in that direction, however. We are talking again about changing the immediate situation of individuals.

I offer the grid only as a kind of taxonomy which may help to clarify what you're doing. If you're working at any of these operational levels, what's your primary goal? Is it change in individuals or change in the immediate milieu or change in the social structure? Being able to answer that will help to clarify what the technology is that you must apply. For example, the technology appropriate to working in a one-to-one individual relationship may not necessarily be the appropriate technology for working in a community. Regardless of what technology you use at the level appropriate to produce individual change, it may not be a useful technology to shape milieu or to change social structures.

The Isomorphic Bias of the Social Scientist

If you examine most mental health theories and try to understand what their implications are for social change you come up with some very interesting observations. For example, Freudian theory is based on an interpretation of society and history that relies heavily on the intrapsychic condition of the individual. In fact, all of the culture according to Freud is a result of repressed infantile sexuality. If one wishes to produce social change, one therefore must produce changes in the dynamic constellation of the individual. The general implication of the Freudian theory is that if you change the individual for the better, he will change society for the better.

If you take the interpersonal theory of psychiatry, you find the same implication; that is, all society is quasi-family. All problems arise, all character, everything is shaped in the original family. If you improve the relationships in the family or in a group or in an organization, you will, then, improve the social structure. That is what I call the isomorphic bias. In other words, a change in one aspect of the situation automatically produces a similar change in the other; if you change an individual for the better he will change society for the better.

Let's turn it around and consider Marx. Marx says if you change society for the better, the individuals in that society will be changed for the better. So, whether you start with the individual and move to society or whether you start with society and move to the individual, most of the social science for the last hundred years has as part of its basic philosophy and theoretical structure an isomorphic bias. I would say that this is a totally unjustified bias and that we have to begin to operate with a different perspective. That is, while there is a relationship between the psychological and social conditions of man, it is not necessarily a one-to-one isomorphic relationship. Once you start with that, you can begin to develop a macropsychology independent of, but related to, the whole body of knowledge contained in what we now have in this country (a micropsychology) which has been the historical orientation of psychology for the last hundred years.

An Alternative: Macropsychology

While related to changes it may produce in the individual, macropsychology does not assume a one-to-one relationship. One can produce a better society with worse individuals or a worse society with better individuals. Once you have that perspective, the means by which you can work with social structures become clear. This is an extremely difficult concept to get people to act upon. Sooner or later when you raise these questions somebody will say, "But aren't you in the long run really working for changed individuals? Isn't it human beings—individuals—who do everything, and aren't you really in the long run working to change individuals?" And my answer is a shocking one: "I'm not interested in individuals. I am interested in social structures and that's what I want to change."

Then the next question is usually: "What's your value system? How can you go ahead and decide you're going to change social structures without some value system?" My answer is that I have looked at human history and have found that there is at least one value that seems to be persistent throughout human history, and perhaps two. And, since these are values that have persisted throughout human history, they offer a fair enough basis on which to operate. These two values are distributive justice and rationality. Those are the two values on which I base any operation to change social structures.

What value does the mentally healthy person have? I would challenge anyone to tell me what mental health is, how they're going to produce it, the relationship between the change in society, and some concept of mental health. I offer you the suggestion that happiness is not as good a value as distributive justice for changing social structures if you want to be a change agent in this country. The mental health movement has little or nothing to offer at the present time. You cannot generate social and political programs on the basis of mental health concepts.

During the period when the blacks first came out for black power in this country, many of the psychologists jumped on board and said, "Yes, we're for black power. Why are we for black power?

Because it will help the blacks achieve psychological autonomy." That is sheer nonsense, which subsequent events have proven. In the first place, the concept of psychological autonomy has nothing to do with the problem of political power. There are people who have political power and have no psychological autonomy. And there are people who have no political power and have a great deal of psychological autonomy. There is not that kind of one-to-one relationship.

Power is as much likely to corrupt a person as it is to enhance him. We know that from the way power operates. It doesn't take a very wise man to make a statement of that kind. I was for black power because I thought it was just. Because I felt the blacks have as much right to be corrupted as the whites, not because of any psychological autonomy or any such mental health reason. There's a concrete example of how two different values lead to doing two different views although we both may support black power. But it's a totally different kind of support.

One of my mentors taught me that the fundamental role of the change agent or somebody interested in social change should be that of helping people to change the society in whatever way they want to change it. Some people say that's a cop-out, but that was his answer. Anybody that wants to be a change agent and is interested in social planning is immediately taking on a whole series of contradictory positions and contradictory situations. For example, what is the role of a change agent in a democratic country? How can you do planning, and can you do planning in a democratic country? Can you do national planning in a country where you're primarily interested in pluralistic development? There are a whole number of issues that are raised once you decide to enter into the area of social planning. And some people will contend that social planning is antidemocratic.

The major dilemma in prevention in mental health is that society is producing casualties faster than we can deal with them. The logical and rational way to deal with it is not to put your finger in the dike, but to build a more formidable dam. On the other hand, you're faced with the humanistic dilemma. What do you do with all the casualties in society that are created because society does not have at the present time enough resources to deal with the prevention problem and the casualty problem at the same time? So you really have a very serious dilemma. What do you do?

Leonard Hassol, a participant in the 1965 Swampscott Conference that launched community psychology, traces the connections between the community mental health movement and a variety of techniques for bringing about social change in communities. In illustrating various strategies for change, such as advocacy, collaboration, and conflict, Hassol examines some of the valued and ethical issues in which social scientists are likely to find themselves involved, particularly the elitist views that are so often unwittingly espoused by those who would try to do good for others.

Chapter 9

FROM MENTAL HEALTH TO SOCIAL CHANGE WITHOUT A PARACHUTE: HOW TO SURVIVE

Leonard Hassol

Allow me to begin with a personal anecdote that can teach us an important truth about working for social change. When I was 13 years old, my maternal grandmother, who was then 92, lived with my family. She had emigrated from Poland as a young woman to escape persecution, had lived in severe poverty for many years, labored in the New York sweatshops, and had borne nine children only to see five of them die in a diphtheria epidemic. But in spite of all that, or maybe because of it, she was a very sturdy, self-reliant old lady whose orthodox religious faith left little room for wishful thinking or self-importance. Only a few things in life really mattered to her: her family, her religion, and whether those dear to her were "making a living." There was, therefore, not much in life that could throw her for a loss. As with many adolescents, however, almost everything was throwing me. I was unhappy about myself, the world, and everything in between. And so one day, after listening to me bitch and moan endlessly about how unhappy I was, my grandmother peered up at me over the top of her bifocals and asked quietly, "So where is it written that *you* must be happy?"

Social scientists are clearly not happy these days. The world doesn't seem to love us anymore. Grants fail, our efforts at social change are scorned. Perhaps, since nowhere is it written that we *must* be happy, a look at how we reached this point of no joy, and what we may have overlooked along the way, will suggest some new beginnings.

In 1965, what has become known as the Swampscott Conference was able to launch the field of community psychology into the world, largely because of two connected situations: (1) The spirit of the times, the zeitgeist, was right. It was the time of the New Frontier and the Great Society, the brief period when the country seemed to have made a commitment to try for social justice. (2) Applied social science types where being invited into the tent. At Swampscott, psychologists such as Bob Reiff and Jim Kelly, or Lou Cohen and Ira Iscoe, were all heavily involved in the Peace Corps, Job Corps, Community Action Programs, Model Cities, all the new wine that seems so sweet to our innocent palates.

Eric Hoffer once said something to the effect: "Give intellectuals everything they want—except power." Well, the social scientists have been kicked out of the tent, the rhetoric has subsided. During that brief reign, however, we did a lot of significant "seat-of-the-pants" experimentation. Much community consultation work has gone on since. The need now is to draw some general principles of social change from all this experience.

Perspectives for Change

Since a professor is known by the concepts he keeps, I hasten to spread before you a three-level schema that has helped me through many noisy and confused events in the world of social change activity. Most of the initial situations with which a client system will ask me to assist fall under the heading of problem solving. If I prove useful at that level, larger issues are presented calling for planned change. And sometimes matters develop that call for activities that can be termed social intervention.

Problem-solving

This is where many of us began to move out of the clinical format and into the early model of group mental health consultation. A specific source of tension exists in a social system, and the consultant is called in to see what can be done. Before this, the tension usually focused around an individual, say a troublesome child in school.

However, I would like to walk you through a more complex and current example that starts as problem solving and then develops opportunities for moving to planned change and social intervention efforts.

There is a high school near me which, in physical terms, is gigantic; 5900 students in one recently constructed building, reputedly the largest public school east of the Mississippi. In terms of equipment and varied educational opportunities it is unsurpassed, but, nevertheless, it has troubles to fit its size. A major social indicator is that on any given day about 1200 students are playing hookey for one reason or another. That is a large number for the community to contend with, especially after it had spent 8 million dollars for the new building. The Superintendent of Schools, a personal friend, asked me to see what I could do to help bring some of the kids back to school.*

Now, with the exception of a focus on an entire high school, this level of problem solving is still typical of consultation as practiced around the country. The standard questions are of the order, Why can't kids read? Why are kids skipping school? And, sometimes, What can we do in the classroom to deal with these issues? The responses that are acceptable to the school people tend to be framed in individualistic terms that keep the "problem" located mostly within the skin of individual students. After hearing the high school principal, house masters, and teachers sing about eight different versions of the old refrain "What's wrong with the kids?" I wanted to yell back, "What's wrong with this place? Why are you generating so many casualties?" Of course you can't do that. The start had to be made where it was hurting them and where they could listen, even though many individuals in the system had intimations that the problem wasn't only the kids. The best version of a response that the school staff could produce was (in that absolutely terrible phrase), "How can we better reach the kids?" My answer at this stage of

_____

* Incidentally, a fascinating commentary on community decision making resides in the reason that such an elephantine structure was erected in the first place. Educational consultants, the faculty, the school superintendent, all inveighed against the plan as an educational horror show; but one man was mightily in favor of it ... the high school football coach who had delivered the state football championship to the city, since the memory of man runneth not to the contrary. This worthy gentleman merely stood up at the crucial city council meeting and pointed out that two smaller high schools would jeopardize the championship by dividing the talent pool from which his adolescent gladiators were drawn. The educational purposes of the new high school were drowned in a rip-tide of municipal blood-lust and patriotism. Any questions about the true sources of power in American communities?

entry into the system was to grit my teeth and say simply, "Let's find out." What I meant by that was a process of gathering information about the way it felt to live in that school, under its particular rules and personnel, from the students, staff, and administrators, My students and I spent eight months designing an interview schedule, getting input from students, teachers, and administrators, and then giving it to a representative sample of the school constituencies. The findings spoke directly to the attendence problem, and many others as well. But at that point further movement required switching to a planned change perspective.

Planned Change

A good portion of the community psychology activity of the 1960s involved planned change. Activities and structures designed to assist client systems cope more effectively with their problems, i.e., Neighborhood Service Centers, organizations in Community Action Programs, and National Training Laboratory training programs, etc. exemplify this trend. For the details of how this is done I refer you to Ronald Lippet's *The Dynamics of Planned Change*, to Donald Klein's *Community Dynamics and Mental Health* (1968), and to Bob Reiff's varied publications in this area (1967, 1968). In the most general terms, planned change efforts focus either on improving the communication patterns and organizational style of a client system or on the creation of new institutional structures for coping with emerging problems. Often a mixture of the two is necessary.

In the high school example just cited, the planned change phase began with an effort to use the survey findings as a lever for moving the several subgroups off the center of their assumptions and preconceptions. The findings were reported back to small groups of teachers, students, and administrators, and were framed in such a way as to highlight the discrepancies between each group's view of the behavior of the others. For example, how does it happen that while teachers believe they are usually fair and evenhanded in their dealings with students, the students believe just the opposite? Discussions of this kind gradually led to consideration of alternative ways of handling the everyday, recurring issues of life at school that were the source of much grief for all three constituencies. The ideas which emerged ranged all the way from better screening techniques for the hiring of teachers who could relate comfortably to adolescents, to more imaginative, less rigid use of space, to inputs from both students and teachers into major policy decision making, etc.

And a final ingredient, one so often forgotten, was an evaluation system designed, not to put the finger on individuals, but rather, to aid in keeping the emerging system responsive to changing conditions.

Social Intervention

With social intervention, we deal more with dreams and possibilities than proven reality, and many would say that we are dealing in grandiosity and pipe dreams. Serious efforts at changing basic societal or institutional arrangements in the interest of solving old social problems or meeting newly emerging social needs are still rare. Even rarer are such efforts consciously thought out in advance by social scientists. The Community Corporation efforts in Cincinnati, or the attempt at community-controlled mental health centers in New York City, both short-lived and funded on soft money (money temporarily supplied by grants or contracts with fixed terms), stand out as singularities from which little generalization is possible. And as long as we look for social intervention at the level of national policy (both examples above ultimately traced back to federal support) we will find none. As Ryan (1969) has noted, American social policy tends to be characterized by an emphasis on short-term goals and an avoidance of long-term planning. Additionally, change sponsored by the federal government tends toward the very slow accretion of new structures, usually brought about by the pragmatic response to a narrow situation, rather than a distinct and well-thought-out plan to deal with a broad issue. There is a long and cancerously ingrained tradition in the United States of *not* having any national policies to deal with major social problems.

We therefore have to get back to potentialities for social intervention, and we probably have to look at the local level for the foreseeable future. To use the high school example, what might a genuine social intervention in that setting look like? One idea would be the creation of an alternative school, a much smaller operation run jointly by students and teachers in which all questions, including curriculum, hiring, and firing, and budget utilization are decided on a community basis. In essence, this would be an alternative to the one huge school, an option for the community to study, to chew over, and to decide if it had any virtues transferrable to the way the large school was run.

This idea of setting up a working demonstration of a new idea is most important; the philosopher Alfred North Whitehead once said that society never merely thinks its way to the solution of social problems; it has to see possible answers acted out, and then it decides whether or not it buys a particular answer. That's been one of the big difficulties that social scientists have had in dealing with government; we approach elected officials with some pretty fancy theoretical arguments, but there's no experience backing us. We ask society to take one hell of a risk. We say, "We'll play the game for you if you give us the chips. We won't live in the new arrangements we're proposing, but we will set them up for you to live in."

I once served as the on-call community psychologist in an alternative high school. Originally, it was created as a place for the kids who were just about to drop out of the main high school, a last hope for "the kids we haven't been able to reach." Now it has a mixed population composed of some of the most achieving students in the high school as well as many turned off young people. It contains 110 students, 8 teachers, many community residents contributing services from time to time, and all of it housed in a former elementary school located in a working-class neighborhood away from the main high school. A few random points will give both the flavor and the challenge of the place.

The first 4 weeks of school are spent in students and staff meeting to decide on what's going to be offered and what the learning format will be. That drives people on the school committee, some parents, and some faculty of the regular high school up the wall. Much effort goes into bringing these skeptics into school and showing them the long-range learning benefits that accrue to students from such an experience.

The activities in the school are very visible to the neighborhood, what with Yoga classes on the front lawn, and other elitist diversions. The average working person did not appreciate this going on in their school. The odd nature of this school was made acceptable by the school offering a service to the community that was really needed, an inexpensive, student-run nursery school for the children of working mothers in the neighborhood. It became the focus for the entire human development component of the high school curriculum, as well as a means of drawing the neighborhood people into the school so they could see what was actually happening.

An alternative social institution of this kind is accommodated by the larger community through a labeling process; since it's deviant from the norm it can be walled off and ignored, if not tolerated. What already exists is the norm. That is the way things should be. Anything different has to go through a lengthy trial by fire to prove itself even though what exists may be doing a terrible job.

We are familiar with this process in the smug challenge thrown at primary prevention programs by clinicians who ask for proof that prevention activities ever helped anybody. Such folks are bewildered and angry when you ask them for the proof that psychotherapy, of any variety, has ever helped anybody. When you've been doing something long enough in a certain way it takes on the status of a revealed truth.

Conflict, Advocacy, Collaboration: Take Your Choice

The categories I've discussed so far neatly describe change activities, but they are merely static descriptions. Let's look at a more dynamic threesome, and let's begin with conflict and competition, concepts which a recent Secretary of the Treasury endorsed as "the rock on which we have built our earthly temple."

Conflict Strategy

Americans generally seem to be addicted to a win-lose view of human affairs. For someone to win, someone else has to lose (or thinks they have to, which amounts to the same thing). Everything, from football to sex, tends to be turned into a win-lose situation. School busing for racial balance has been cast in that light; labor–management bargaining is seen this way; and the funding of human service programs is certainly fought out on those lines. I am quite persuaded, however, that conflict can be a most creative approach to social problems. Very little would change without some degree of conflict and competition. And when people depend on their own resources, as they must in many conflict situations, success leads to an enhanced sense of autonomy and power, which leads to accepting new challenges. The success of active confrontational tactics advocated by Saul Alinsky is evidence of how effective a conflict strategy can be when skillfully pursued. Teaching people how to fight for their rights and needs is a very legitimate role for one breed of change agent.

Of course, the Alinsky version of conflict strategy is an extreme position that deliberately seeks polarization of the issues. More often a kind of compromise, or more accurately, a synthesis, is implicit in conflict situations since each party, simply as a matter of good strategy, needs to see the other position more clearly and with reduced stereotyping. A good arbitrator will capitalize on this characteristic, working toward clarification and specificity and away from simplified agendas which lead toward the extreme "I win, you lose" hang up.

Advocacy

Advocacy is a special version of conflict strategy in which a decision is made that certain victims are either too far victimized to be able to help themselves, or that the skills required simply cannot be taught within the time or resources available to accomplish a desired result. Therefore, you do the job on your own. A brief example will make this clear.

A group of activist law students at the University of Chicago in the early 1960s decided to tackle the issue of substandard housing conditions in the ghetto slums of the South Side. Preliminary investigation revealed that perpetuation of violations of the housing codes was due to a web of interlocking factors: hidden absentee ownership, wholesale bribery of building inspectors and politicians, indifference of the mortgage-holding banks because of the high interest rates produced by these slum mortgages. The students went to work on several fronts. They dug through layers of legal disguise to locate the true owners, who were some of the wealthier people in town, and publicized their slumlord status. They catalogued a broad sample of the housing code violations and sent them to the insurance companies which held the insurance on the buildings. The insurance companies, as a matter of self interest, told the banks that all insurance would be canceled if the violations were not corrected promptly, and then, of course, the banks told the slumlords that the mortgages would be foreclosed if the insurance lapsed. Almost immediately most of the major violations were corrected. The residents didn't even know anyone was in their corner until the carpenters showed up. Here was a direct advocacy strategy in which a pure value stance was taken to the effect that certain people ought to win and others deserved to lose.

Collaboration Strategy

Collaboration strategy tends to appeal to many in the middle-class. It may be worth a passing notice that change agents who tend toward conflict and advocacy positions, such as Bob Reiff or Saul Alinsky, came out of working-class origins and severe depression-years experiences, while collaboration practitioners like Don Klein, or even myself, emerged from more sheltered, less traumatic early backgrounds.

Well, collaboration is a strategy that attempts to find grounds on which divergent groups can come together in their mutual self-interest. The concept of superordinate goals, goals which several groups desire but none can achieve on its own, underlies much of this point of view. The operational group that has been most persistent in developing collaboration techniques has been the National Training Laboratory (NTL) Institute. Starting with Kurt Lewin and growing under the guidance of people like Ronald Lippet, Kenneth Benne, and Warren Bennis, NTL pioneered the development of human relations training on the one hand, and organizational analysis on the other. Taken together these approaches account for both the interpersonal and the environmental forces that either help or hinder desired change processes. They make it possible to tackle many problems in the full complexity of their human and organizational interaction.

Again, an example is needed to give reality to these abstractions. A few years ago I was part of an NTL group working for the Model Cities Administration on the creation of health delivery teams in model cities areas across the country. This involved bringing together representatives of competing minority groups, the business establishment, city hall, the medical community, and the residents of the model cities areas who are going to be trained as members of health delivery teams. NTL approached this with a detailed collaborative strategy based on human relations training approaches.

Our first effort in Philadelphia failed miserably. Even before the meeting began, we were drowned in hostility from angry blacks, Chicanos, and Mayor's representatives for that matter, all of whom resented terribly the imposition of a whole series of federal stereotypes as to what was wrong with the health system in the ghettos and how it should be corrected. It turned out that the major sponsor, the Department of Housing and Urban Development (HUD), had tried to deal with these same groups in the past and had met the same reception. Constrained by congressional, budgetary, and political pressures, HUD administrators hoped without ever telling us that NTL might be able to get the client groups to "be reasonable." We went back to HUD and insisted that for the next city on the list, San Francisco, some top HUD officials would be present to (1) apologize for the fact that they had not been able to include the local people in the initial planning, and (2) be present for the entire workshop and attentive to ways in which the procedures of the bureaucracy might be modified to respond to the desires of local residents and officials.

Eventually we did get to the point whère we could apply our collaborative approach. Many of the competing groups began to see the value for each of them in combining forces to achieve some new kinds of health delivery systems that were badly needed by their constituents. In short, with the proper attention to the political and communication barriers inherent in such complex social environments, you can get people who are in competition to collaborate if there are superordinate goals which can be made clearly visible.

Commingling of Categories

These neat categories I've presented obviously get mixed up and lose their conceptual purity. When labor and management face each other, the question of wages is mostly a win-lose situation, but while fighting over that they had better keep in mind that there are other issues on which they *can* collaborate without loss for either side; push the conflict issues too hard and they dirty the field for the collaborative possibilities on such things as seniority, fringe benefits, etc.

I want to present an example of a mixed situation to illustrate how one must be ready to shift the approach as new conditions unfold in the flux of real community change efforts. The chairman of the mental health board serving the city of Attleboro, Massachusetts, asked me if the students in my community psychology field-work program could be of assistance in a long-range project aimed at "improving children's services" in the community. After some clarifications and defining of responsibilities, I assigned a team of three responsible and presentable students to work with the board for an academic year.

They began by designing and conducting a survey of all the agencies who were actually supplying children's services in the catchment area, something that had never been done before. Along with a lot of new and useful information, they turned up a vast area of conflict among the various service agencies; issues of territoriality, claims on limited and shrinking resources, rigid professional guild definitions of who was qualified to do what, and varied political conflicts among agencies who, on the surface at least, were all committed to improving children's services. When their initial report made it apparent that the student team had become the resident experts on the true nature and quality of children's services in the area, many of the agencies tried to co-opt them into becoming a weapon in the battle. Most difficult of all, the area mental health board, our original client, also began efforts to hook the students in as their operatives in the conflict. The message was that the board, in efforts to maximize its control over children's services, wanted the students to reveal whatever politically embarassing information about other agencies they had accumulated during the survey. Of course, it wasn't said as crassly as that, but the meaning was clear. And since the area board was our entree into a very worthwhile enterprise, well, what indeed do you do?

It was also true that the students saw the area board as the best equipped, most representative group to act as the umbrella organization, so it was tempting to simply help them fight on their terms.

After a lot of discussion with the students, we decided to try to demonstrate to the area board that it was not in *their* interest for us to comply with the request. The student team went back with the following message in mind: "If we were to do as you ask, to reveal this kind of information, some of which we have, though far less than you seem to think we have, we would quickly be discredited in the rest of the professional community, people would know where it came from. We could no longer operate effectively as outside, disinterested students working to improve area children's services. You would lose, and probably everyone else would lose."

We finally settled into more of an advocacy role than we had originally had. We decided to present ourselves to all the agencies and say that the best role for the students was to be advocates for the children of the area, and collaborators with the agencies in fighting the children's services funding battles going on in the state legislature. That battle was in the interest of all concerned and was a superordinate goal.

What emerged was a unique decision to allow the students, using the resources of all the agencies, to recruit, organize, and train a citizens' group who would, in turn, conduct a community education program about the needs of children, leading, hopefully, to a citizens' lobby capable of exerting direct pressure on the legislature. That was the model agreed upon, and it went forward with moderate success.

Colleagues have asked, "Why did you, an outsider, do this job—as opposed to someone in social welfare or social service in the community?" It seems to me that what's lacking in almost all American communities is someone who has the sanction to be the "thinker" for the entire community, someone who can look at the whole system and suggest where it is functioning well, where it is falling down, what might be done, and by what values these judgements can be made. Such questions are almost never asked; instead you merely get ad hoc proposals: "Let's fight heart disease this year, cancer the next," etc. Salted into the mix are issues of bureaucratic and individual survival, and what the mayor thinks will get him votes, all of which makes it difficult for anybody to take on the role of applied town intellectual. Someone from outside the struggle may be given the chance to try or, as friends have suggested, enough rope to hang himself. But that is a risk you have to take if you want a piece of the action.

Further Permutations

Traditional psychological practices (in the instance just cited, interviewing, survey research, and adult education) can be used in the service of new social goals, and this activity can take place under the aegis of traditional service settings. The local community mental health center, especially in rural areas, will usually contain the only available personnel trained to think systematically and methodologically about assisting communities to define social problems and to experiment with new solutions. If the staff of the center can accept such a role redefinition, they will find many possibilities for participation in social change efforts in their own backyard. To illustrate this point I will list a few of the things we undertook during the years I directed the community consultation service at the South Shore Mental Health Center, Quincy, Massachusetts:

> Training and collaborating with a group of mothers on welfare in the development of a politically effective voter registration drive in the slum areas of the city.
> In collaboration with a group of public school teachers, the development and implementation of a behavioral science curriculum for grades K–12 oriented to primary prevention.
> Development and training of a group of clergymen able to identify, train, and supervise a network of crisis counselors within their congregations. Examples are parents who had coped successfully with the experience of raising a retarded child acting as counselors for other parents just facing that same crisis, or successfully married couples serving as resources for newly married couples facing the early strains of marriage.

Acting as consultants, proposal writers, and policy advisors to the Mayor on matters concerning social programming, obtaining federal funds for human service programs, etc.

Manipulation and Social Change

Finally, I'd like to say a word about the ethics of social change activity, and more specifically, the question of manipulation and free choice. As far as I know, the person who's done the best thinking about this problem is Herb Kelman. In his book *A Time to Speak*, Kelman (1968) says there is no possibility of avoiding some degree of manipulation in social change activity. That being the case, the only remedy is to make clear to your clients that some degree of manipulation is taking place, but also, that your efforts are designed to be self-limiting. You are trying to assist your clients to become aware of manipulation and, finally, to be able to function without outside manipulation. In effect, they share the risks with you since you state ahead of time what the risks are.

The several strategies I've discussed have different implications for the lives of the people who will be affected by change. It's perfectly within the right of a professional to analyze a situation and decide what strategy, or mix of strategies, would accomplish a given outcome. But it's also the absolute right of the people whose lives will be changed to decide if they want to let you go ahead and do it. If you don't like their decision, if they opt for a strategy which you cannot conscientiously accept, then you retire from the scene.

This is especially difficult to carry out when there is a third party present who has both a firm concept of what needs to be done and the funds to pay for having it done. An article by Mills and Kelly (1972) about intervention in Mexican Indian villages is an excellent case in point. The social scientists involved simply accepted the Mexican government's dictate that all Indian tribes had to be removed from their pastoral state. The position could easily be rationalized that it is better for these people to be in the mainstream of life than not, they'll be free of disease, their children will be educated, etc. The fact that a whole culture and pastoral way of life would be destroyed in the process is a consequence that *we* will decide if *they* can bear.

Social Values

The people doing the many things alluded to above, the agents of change, seem to be endowed with a high level of restless and perfectionistic energy, a kind of brash, perhaps arrogant self-confidence that moves them to decide that various social arrangements need to be altered. This elitist tendency can be controlled if our field can agree on some broad social values which ought to inform our efforts.

Let me conclude by briefly describing three broad value categories which appeal to me:

1. *The value of sustaining life.* All objects and activities that help satisfy peoples' basic requirement for food, shelter, healing, survival, and personal meaning are life-sustaining goods that society ought to nurture and protect. To the extent that the pursuit of other objects and activities threatens these goods, society ought to be in a posture of resistance and change.

2. *The value of esteem.* This refers to every person's sense that he or she is a being of worth, that they deserve a fundamental respect and that, therefore, they are not being used as an object or tool by others for the attainment of purposes and goals to which they have not given their informed consent.

3. *The value of freedom.* This is a most vexing, but eternally beckoning ideal which probably can never be fully reached, but which, at the very least, implies an extended range of choice for societies and their members. Such choice must take place against a background of awareness, awareness of the nature and range of the real options, of the unavoidable constraints, and of the consequences, as best they can be foreseen, flowing from each choice. In short, rational selection must be possible free of deception, coercion, or manipulation by the state, corporations, or individuals.

Whether or not this set of social values wins your assent, I agree with Bob Reiff and others who suggest that we must develop some consensus on social values before we can decide on the social goals we wish to support and the constituents in whose interests we will work. Without such guiding values our work will always seem improvised, and be subject to co-optation by groups and interests who *do* know what kind of world they want.

HUMAN SERVICES DELIVERY IN THE CONTEXT OF POLITICS AND TRADITION

One message that comes from the chapters thus far and is reinforced in those that follow is that we Americans are able to devise and sustain very complex solutions to what are inherently quite simple individual human problems. Our public and private health services are complex and costly and variously effective. But are they efficient and accessible and are they open to change? Our family assistance services are even more complex and they vary from state to state. They too are variously effective, but are they efficient and accessible and open to change? Our services on behalf of those who are mentally ill in a technical sense or who are just chronically unhappy and functioning below their capabilities are many and complex and often in competition with one another. They too are producing results, but are they efficient, accessible, and open to change?

Most of the answers to the questions of efficiency and openness to change come out in the negative. Costs per client in most helping services continue to rise along with the numbers of clients. Measures of effectiveness continue to be elusive (and so they deny any precise or quantitative answer to the question of efficiency) and virtually all ways of delivering assistance to those in need resist change, with the few exceptions of those whose financial base is so poor that they change from a state of presence to one of absence.

Why does all of this come about and why does it continue? It is one of the problems as well as one of the blessings of the democratic form of government that legislators and service agency administrators respond to the constituencies that they hear from. The creation of the Administration on Aging and the National Institute on Aging at the federal level, and the rash of local Area Agencies on Aging is the most conspicuous recent example of this. Audible constituencies thus can create organizations dedicated to good service, including often some services which can be obtained through already existing means. People in organizations also typically become dedicated to maintaining their own jobs, which often leads to major investments in keeping the organization alive, draining off resources that otherwise might go toward the officially expected human service. When this behavior occurs in public service agencies, it is called bureaucratic fence building, or by other opprobrious names. When it occurs in private enterprise it is called natural competition for product improvement or for the proper pursuit of profit.

But philosophical issues aside for the moment, the democratic process permits, even encourages, the development of service systems that quickly evolve their own reasons for being and which resist change in the ways in which they become accustomed to doing the proper and good things they were set up to do. Fortunately, also, the democratic process makes possible the constant and occasionally successful assault on the "way things are done."

Change is not out of the question; it is just difficult. To close a tax-supported mental hospital, even one whose malefits clearly exceed its benefits to patients, is not a simple managerial task. It may affect the jobs of a thousand people and the lives of their additional thousands of family members and nearby merchants who depend in part on them, not to mention the community's tax base so dear to all political and economic interests. And what state legislator wants to risk unemployment and the loss of legislators' perquisites just in the name of efficiency in a service whose efficiency *can't* be proved anyway? And what service agency manager wants to see his organization smaller and risk a degrading of his own job-description and position rating in the interest of a consolidation of "his" service with another?

Is there a solution to the problem of overlapping services, to the "nightmare of categorical services and conflicting eligibilities"? Perhaps a better question is: *Should* there be a clean, clear, and final solution to such problems? The negative answer to this form of the question implies that in a democratic society one of the obligations of membership is to tolerate ambiguity and the complexity and competitiveness of service that is generally inherent in the democratic mystique, to be willing to constantly struggle for solutions and be willing to settle intermittently for the less than desired while continuing to struggle, on the faith that the system does afford the possibility for change, and (perhaps grudgingly) to respect or at least to admit the legitimacy of other people's preferred ways and their claims to autonomy. We hold that this is the way change must come about in our ways of inventing, managing, and changing systems for delivering human services so long as we choose to do those things within the govenmental framework we have inherited.

But, one should finallly ask, does this mean that we must be endlessly tolerant of waste, duplication, and inefficiency, in the process, and simply stand idly by in the faith that things will automatically work out for the best in the long run? Certainly not. And the reason for it is that we do not live in a society with limitless resources, that we do live in a society with an unequal distribution of power and opportunity, that we do espouse, however unclearly at times, the belief that each person should have an opportunity to develop his capabilities to some satisfying extent, if not to some imaginary maximum of potential. Given these conditions and beliefs, public policy does assign a high value to the goal of meeting basic human needs, a value higher than the goal of tolerating "needs" of organizations (public or private), and thus to continue to encourage service system change and to demand some measure of accountability in the meeting of those basic needs.

Thus democracy, when operating reasonably well, is a means for providing for constant evolution of social forms and for the fostering of relatively peaceful change and for providing conditions that will make possible continuing human development.

Most of us are familiar with the distinction made between federal, state, and local levels of government. Each has a distinct perspective, but there is no doubt that the buck stops at the local level. There is also no doubt that the county is a critical form of local government. Like prospectors searching for minerals, the commissioners and their staffs prospect the various terrains of federal and state legislation for natural resources their constituents need. Like captains of the old windjammers, they have to readjust their sails and shift cargo to meet changes in the direction of superordinate winds. And like the Biblical prophets, they see the needs of the people, their foibles, the arbitrariness of Caesar and his proclamations, and bend to the task. Typical or not, Commissioner Spearly's account gives us an insight into the life and thought of an elected county official in rural American. It shows how it is possible to tie together the many strands of finance, bureaucracy, tradition, political influence and human decency in looking after people's physical and emotional well being.

Chapter 10

HOW AN ELECTED OFFICIAL SEES COMMUNITY MENTAL HEALTH AT ITS APPLICATION POINT, OR, GETTING THE WORK DONE

Grove A. Spearly, Sr.

I am not going to give you a political talk. But I am going to weave some politics into this because it is part of the landscape. First of all, in politics, any individual who wants to move has got to be very strong. He's got to be dedicated and believe in his convictions, and be willing to work for these convictions.

I realize that there's a lot of people, especially after Watergate, who mistrust politicians. They think they're a bunch of bureaucrats, and they're just out to get the dollar, and so forth. That's not so. You can be just as honest in politics as you can in any other profession, because there are good people in politics, as well as bad ones; we're very fortunate in having good ones in Centre County. People will vote for the man who produces. I'm not ashamed to be called a politician, and I'm proud of my accomplishments.

Honesty and fairness is what counts. Of course, that applies to any profession. There's no substitute for right. I've always said that. Don't be persuaded by somebody who's going to pass some money under the table. I encountered one person who, if I'd been strong enough, I would have bodily thrown him out. He wanted to give me $5000 if I'd turn my back on something that was going to cost the County somewhere between $20 and $50 thousand. I didn't know how much exactly; I wasn't smart enough to know. But I was smart enough to know what was on the specs of what was going on in the building program we were doing. And if the specs were wrong, I couldn't help that. But they were going to be what the specs were and nothing else.

Sometimes it's very hard to determine right from wrong. But if you stand by your conviction of what's right, and make a decision, you stick to it. There should be no turning around ten minutes after it's made when somebody comes in or calls you on the telephone and gives you hell because you may have made the wrong decision. You can say, "Well, I'm very sorry but the decision is made." Taxpayers always have the chance of voting you out if you don't do the proper job.

Another thing I'd like to say: First thing of all, before you get anywhere, you've got to be a registered voter and vote. This is the way we get good government. We're not about to get good government, we're not about to get good services unless we register and vote, and I don't care how a person registers; I was always more or less nonpartisan in that I was never a party politician. Being a Democrat in a Republican county with 8000 votes against you, you don't go out and try to slap the opposition in the face. You try to win them over.

Now I want to give you a little background on the county commissioners: how you get to be one and what happens when you get there. Four people are nominated at a primary election, two from each party. Then after the primary, there's a run-off in the general election, and the top three people are the winners. You always have a majority and a minority commissioner. Of course, in this county it's very seldom that they have a majority of Democratic commissioners. It has happened. If the right people run, it can happen, because, again, I have a lot of faith in the people, and that includes a lot of faith in young people. If people get out and are really interested in somebody, and he tries to do the job and you study him and think that he's the person, you think, "Well, I'm going to vote for that man because I think he's all right." I've made some mistakes too. I've voted for people that I thought were all right, and it turned out they weren't all right. This is something we all do. The person that never made a mistake in life never got very far. Of course, I make plenty of them.

Then, of course, after you're elected, the commissioners elect a chairman. The chairman of the board is the person who gets the highest number of votes, or the other two members can elect him. I was a minority commissioner, and I had the highest votes of any of them in the county. But I didn't want to be chairman, though in fact, some people insisted. Some of my Republican friends that helped me get where I was insisted that they were going to make me chairman of the board. I said no, I don't want to be chairman of the board.

I'll give you reasons why. When you are chairman of the board you have to accept all of the motions. When I was sitting back there as a minority commissioner, I made the decisions. Any time they weren't together, I voted. I made a lot of motions. I think if you look at the records that my batting average was about 90 percent. I always said if I got 90, I'd give the other two commissioners 10 percent because I thought that was a pretty good batting average. But you don't go into a meeting fighting, ripping mad. You have to be very cool and calm and collected. The other thing you do is lay all your groundwork before you make your moves. It's like playing baseball or any sport or anything you do. Make sure you're right, and then when you make your move, stick to it.

Now all of this relates to human services because it relates to people. They have 34 different programs in the county commissioners' offices. The tax assessment is one. Of course, you know that you can't operate unless you get taxes. You have a veterans' administrator. There are many programs—just about everything—liquid fuel, planning, prison, and so forth.

A Little on Planning and Budgeting

I have tried to get the housing we need so badly in this area—low-cost housing. I was unfortunate enough, I guess, to be with colleagues who didn't care about low-cost housing. One of them was a real estate man both terms that I served as county commissioner. So they didn't want any part of low-cost housing because that was going to cut in on them. But finally, we got the first step. They said we'd have to have planning to get the housing. So we got planning started. Finally (and I don't mean that I was the whole commission, but I want to get across to you people how things are done) we did get a housing authority appointed. I think there will be some outcomes.

But the problem in planning is this: you have to plan no matter what you're going to do, but you've got one problem with planning in our county. It takes too long. I want to see something done. I want to see the brick and mortar. You know, you can plan for a year or a year and a half, and when you get through planning, it's obsolete. So you start over and you plan again. Really, we need housing in the worst kind of way in Centre County. Everytime it seems that somebody throws the wrench in it. Then, I think, it's because of the pressure that's been brought by real estate men. I was always strong enough as a commissioner that I could stand almost any pressure anybody put on me. When they called me up and raised hell over the telephone, and I would take it if it was coming to me, but if it wasn't coming to me, they got it back in about the same fashion that they tried to give it to me.

We also have certain programs that are mandated in the country; for instance, the Child Welfare Service. These things are mandated by the legislature, and they've got to be carried out. We have the skilled nursing unit for the medically indigent at Centre Crest which now they don't call the County Home; they call it a skilled nursing care facility. We have the MH-MR which you people are familiar with, Veterans' Affairs, and the State Agriculture Extension. You'd wonder why we get mixed up in agriculture extension. Well, this has been an act of legislation whereby the county agent is supported—his office, his staff, and certain supplies—by appropriations from the county commissioners. That's how this comes about.

Then we have programs that are not voluntary but are optional. We've got Community Action, Homemakers' Service, Information Referral Service, and that is something that is very important, because we never had it, and I think in time they may be able to do a good job. They haven't proved to me that they did the job that I wanted done. Then we have the Adult Foster Home Care, Meals on Wheels, and so forth.

This adult foster home care is one that was tied in with our nursing home facilities in the county. We would find a person living in their own home who was not able to take care of their own work, but they really weren't a person who should be institutionalized. So we would find someone who could use the money to care for this person. It might be a lady living by herself, or it might be her and her husband. They could use this money. Of course, these homes were investigated by our staff. We put them there, and they lived very happily. The environment was different. You institutionalize a person and that's the worst thing. Then these people thought: we've got some reimbursement from the public assistance, and they mostly all get Social Security checks so that helped support them. Of course, the state set the amount of money that we had to pay for their care.

To give you some idea of what the human service budget is in Centre County, it is $2.25 million. Ten years ago, when I was county commissioner, our total budget was a little more than $900,000. Now you can see what has happened with the inflationary period. The MH-MR budget is $850,000 for Centre County. Now there is reimbursement from the state and federal government. The county only has to provide 10 percent of this.

A Bit of History

I'm going to take you back and try to bring you up to where we are with some of these things. For instance, how did you take care of the poor 50 years ago? They had overseers of the poor who were elected by the electors in his voting district. Then when somebody needed something, they'd call the overseer of the poor, and of course he would see that they got a doctor if someone was sick. He would see that they got groceries. He would see that they got coal—they didn't have electricity back in those days—or anything that they really needed. Then they would put these people in institutions. Sometimes they called them poor homes. Not all the townships had poor homes, but they would purchase their service.

Today we have a facility to take care of these people in Centre Crest. That's a nursing home with 225 beds, and it still isn't large enough. The budget is $1.5 million to maintain the home.

The first county home was built in 1939; it was mandated by the state. The county commissioners had to build it. They were called county homes or poor houses then at that time. The three commissioners were fine men. They built it because the pressure was on; it was mandated; they had to build it. They never got reelected simply because the people were not educated to what was coming and what direction we moved.

We've come a long way. In this facility we have today things that people hadn't thought of even ten years ago, like physical therapy treatment.

Admission to Centre Crest is by caseworkers who go out and visit people. We may have 50 people on the list, and they admit 51 because they think that the 51st person, after they went over all of them, may be the one that really deserves it more than the other people do. I think the best operation we had in Centre County was our Centre Crest facilities, because we definitely kept politics out of it. We let those people run it. We let them hire the people they wanted to hire, do what they wanted to do, and we took their recommendations. We didn't always agree with them, but when they came in with a budget and explained what they wanted, and if we thought it was fair, there was no problem. When they started in 1930, they only had 80 beds, so you can see we have come quite a way.

Let's get into mental retardation. In those earlier days they would just institutionalize people. They would just put the mentally retarded into an institution, where they were just simply forgotten about. I know one instance where a man was in for 32 years. I finally got him back in a home here through his daughter. People were put away and forgotten about. When they wanted to put somebody in an institution, somebody who was mentally disturbed or violent, they would go through the county commissioners to do this. The reason they went through the county commissioners is because the people who could pay, paid; it might cost the county commissioners $3 a day to take care of someone who did not have anything, in an institution. It might cost the person that had the money $6 a day. I'm just using that as an example. Whereas, if they would admit them through the county, it would be cheaper and then they would reimburse the county.

Today the theory is, as I'm sure you all well know, that we want to deinstitutionalize people and keep them in the community. That's where they should be, in the community, where there are all kinds of volunteers. People in the communities can work more closely. They can help. When you get into a state institution, there's very little help.

The big problem with our mental health and mental retardation resources in Centre County is lack of experience. They're long on theory but very short on experience. I'm not an expert in mental health, and I hope you understand that. I watch and read and try to keep abreast of everything that's going on as I always have done ever since I've been in public office. I see today that they're trying to get their intake and case management service unit changed and put it directly under the MH/MR board. That's really where it belongs, because, before they were contracting the intake and case management services which was really very expensive. Of course you get into the different agencies, and they all have their little empires. For example, when they come into the county commissioner's office and want money, you'd be surprised at how each agency tries to prove it is so much better than the other agencies. You've got to be impartial. You've got to weigh these things and make your decisions.

Staffing

The problem that we have with mental health at the time, as I see it, is the problem of the professional staff. The professional staff we hire in Centre County is paid a lot more than any county commissioner ever gets, but they don't catch any of the hell that the county commissioner catches. I've always said that qualified professionals must have some job security. I never like to see anybody who was really a go-getter in the position he had and did a good job lose their job just because they didn't have the right striped shirt on, or because they were Republican or Democrat. I think it's a very serious mistake. So in order to get around that, they decided that we would put people under civil service.

This is fine, but it also has a terrific effect on people's attitude towards their jobs. They feel, "Well, I'm under civil service, and you can't do anything to me. I'm here for a long time." So people are not as dedicated as they would be if they had competition for the position they're holding. With competition, they think, "Well, I'll do the job. If I don't do it, there might be somebody else to step in and take my position."

Commissioners are Busy People

As I said before, the commissioners get calls. They know who Spearly is, but they don't know who's working under him. If they do know who's working under them, they feel, "I voted for Spearly; he'll get action. I'm not going to talk to some department head or someone because he's going to brush me off." That's the feeling of the electorate. You don't change them. You've got to take care of their problems. You can turn it over to the person who's to take care of them, but you're going to get the telephone calls any hour of the night. It doesn't matter. I never lied to anybody, but finally (it took me a long time) I got Mrs. Spearly to answer the telephone between 6:00 and 7:30 in the evening, while I was having dinner and watching the news, to say that I was out and would be back at 9 o'clock. Then I would take the call. Otherwise I never could sit up to a meal that I didn't get a telephone call.

Some Examples of Problems in Social Services That a County Commissioner Has to Handle

I'll start off with an example that relates to the human services—public assistance. We had a young man whom I got a call from. (I received the calls because most of the people knew that when I got a call they'd get some action, maybe not what they wanted, but some action would be taken immediately. I was on the job all the time. The other commissioners had other interests and weren't always in the office.) This man had nothing to eat in the house and was in a very bad financial situation. We investigated, or had our man investigate it. I put the information in the right place. He came back and said that this man wasn't dismissed and he can't draw unemployment. And in the case I'm referring to the man said, "I was dismissed. I didn't quit." Anyhow, the story was that he couldn't get employment. So we discussed this, and the people came back to me and said, "We're gonna give this fellow a job. We can use him. We need an orderly at Centre Crest. So we won't give him anything unless he earns it—works for it." So they got an affidavit, we gave him the job, and he went to the public assistance office. The public assistance office said, "We're sorry but that caseworker isn't in today." That caseworker isn't in today! And this is the civil service tie-in! You know how far that man had to travel? He had to travel 60 miles because Centre County is one of the large counties in the area. That's 30 miles one way and 30 miles back to get to another appointment a week or so later. You know when you need something today you need it today. You don't need it next week or a month from now. And this is where I think that sometimes they get too professional. Don't get me wrong; I'm for professionals. But I've found that they sit in their office and make an appointment for the next day or something and maybe it should have been taken care of last night. Sometimes they'll put it off for a couple weeks. I never believe in political patronage. I believe strictly on a merit system. If a person's doing a good job, he should stay; if he's not, he should move on.

Back in 1937 (I'm sure you're all familiar with this) a Social Security Act was passed in Pennsylvania which created a Department of Public Assistance. This took the county commissioner clean off the hook from having to provide any services for the poor people outside of (now) maintaining a home for them. But while in their home, if they needed financial help, they went to Public Assistance. You'd be surprised at the amount of people who would call or come to see me and say they didn't have anything in their house to eat. Of course all rules were made to bend. Some arrangement was always made. Maybe I would call up Centre Crest and ask if they could give them some food to tide them over. We weren't in a position to give anybody money, but we never let anybody go hungry. These are things when you get right close to home is where you put it together, and that's where you get the action.

The problems, the rules, the regulations, as I said, are made to bend. But the bureaucrats are very rigid on this. They don't want to bend anything. And they don't have really the picture of the person.

I had a call one day. I think one of the most important things as you go out in life is to know who you're talking to when you're talking to somebody on a problem. It's very important because if a problem comes up and you're called upon to act—to solve this problem—you must always make sure the information you've got is correct.

I'll give you an example. A lady called me one day from Snow Shoe. She was telling me about a case where another lady was living by herself, and she thought she needed help and might have to be put into a nursing home. I knew who the lady was that called me, her financial standing, her husband, and that they were people of means. I knew they were people that wouldn't just call you on the telephone and give you some wrong information. And this lady says, "I'm passing this on. I think this lady's in need." And I said we'll take care of it.

So I called and asked the investigator, the caseworker, and a nurse to go visit this lady. They did it right away, within the next day or so. They came back and told me that they had found that this lady needed corrective shoes. She seemed to have some problems with her feet. She also needed probably an electric stove and an oil burner put in her home; this would be very helpful since she was living on public assistance. I said that if that's all it takes, and we can keep her out of the nursing home and she can be happy in her home, this would be fine. So they proceeded. They got a stove donated to them; they bought an oil burner; they hooked up some valves for the tank. And one of the professional people that works for the county went right out there and hooked it up, seeing that this lady was taken care of.

So what happens when the DPA visits the home? They had allotted in her check four dollars for a boy to get wood and carry it in. So they cut the four dollars off because she didn't need it anymore because she had an oil burner. Anybody with any good judgement knows that it costs more for oil than it does for wood. Now this is the kind of situation where judgements are not used. Every case is different. You've got to use good judgement.

I got a call one evening. Again I knew who the lady was that was calling me. She says that "We have a neighbor that's freezing. There's no heat in the house. I've been over to visit and something has to be done. I'm trying to keep a check on this elderly lady and something has to be done, because if something isn't done, we'll probably have to get her in the county home, Centre Crest." And I said, "Do you know what kind of a stove she needs?" She said, "Yes." I said, "Okay. Where can we get this stove?" and she told me. She said that she'd even gone and checked on the stove but didn't have the money to buy it. So I called the firm where this lady said that she could get the stove. And I said "You get a stove up there this evening." And I described the stove that they wanted. He said, "Yeah, they'd looked into it." And I said, "Get the stove up there and get heat in that house in the next two hours. I want heat in that house." He said, "Okay, it'll be done."

A week or so later we get the bill for the stove. And one of my colleagues, a county commissioner, said to me, "Why are we buying stoves?" I said, "Because I bought that stove. That's why we're buying a stove. It's cheaper for us to buy that stove than to put that poor old soul in an institution." And I said, "She's going to stay in her home."

Now these are cases that you never think of. With all the agencies that I'm speaking about that we have for mental health and things, when it gets right down to it, they're involved more with the county commissioners than anybody else.

I think some counties do go to the extreme of playing politics for even admitting people to homes. If you know the right person, you can get them in and things like that. They'll do their admitting and all that. We had a policy that if they had so much money they could go to another nursing home. And when their money got low, we never sold a home. Instead, we put a judgment on it. That was fair, because it wasn't right for taxpayers of Centre County to pay for this person's keep in our nursing home when the family wouldn't even help. If a child or children wouldn't help their mother or father, we felt it was our duty. We took care of them; we never sold their homes unless there was somebody tried to pull some fraud; and there's always fraud.

We have an awful lot of duplication and waste, and yet it's not being met the way that I feel it should be met. I think agencies often work against other agencies. Like the case of the lady who needed the oil burner. Anything you do you've got to use good judgment and horse sense, and, as I said, the rule will bend.

Again the agencies will come back and say, "Well, maybe we don't have it in the budget." I got things that we never had in the budget, but they had to be taken care of. I'm speaking of the different agencies and programs that say, "Well, we don't have that in the budget so we just don't take care of it."

It seems to me that since the state has come up with so much money for programs, every individual group's going out and trying to get a hold of some of this money to do something with it. But they have never built a facility to put people like alcoholics and drug abusers in to try to rehabilitate them. You can spend all kinds of money, but I think, when you get down to it, you also should have a place to rehabilitate them. And you may have to institutionalize them for a short time, but we're very lax there.

I had a case with a man who was an alcoholic who was calling me frequently. If I got one telephone call, I got 50 telephone calls. This went on for a period of about two years. I knew the gentleman. We got him in Centre Crest and tried to get him straightened up there. When we had him straightened up, we put him out in a foster home. Because he was a meatcutter, we got him a job with a man who was a butcher. So he was doing so well. We told the butcher to keep the booze away from him. If he found any booze, he would have troubles. "It's all right to give him a bottle of beer or something to drink, but don't give him a bottle of booze," we said. We were so proud that somebody would take this man, and here we had solved all the problems that had been going on for so long.

One night he went on a rampage and busted up the furniture in the foster home. Of course he was thrown out in the street again. He went back to the community where he had been before. I started getting the telephone calls again. This time I tried to get mental health to do something: "Isn't there some way we can do something?" And they said, "Well, we'll check it."

He would sleep in automobiles, and they were afraid of fire. He smoked, you know, and he'd get in the garage. He'd sleep in the fireplaces. He didn't have a bed to sleep in. This went on for two years. They finally got him in for a hearing. Finally I went up and testified at the hearing because I knew the man for 35 or 40 years. I thought we had everything all fixed up, and at the end of the hearing the recommendation was to try to get him dried out, put him in an institution. All of a sudden he was back in the community again. Now that case went on and on. Here's a sick person who needs help.

This is what I was speaking about. No matter how many agencies you have, God, if you don't take action and do something—get something accomplished—there's no use having the agencies just sitting around.

I had another case that I want to give you as an example. And there's a lot of these cases in Centre County! I got a call one morning right after I got into the office. And I always was a pretty early riser. I'd always get in the office about 7:30 so I could get a lot of work done before the traffic started to move. I get this call from a man, and he said to me, "My neighbor is up here. He's laying in a room. He's paralyzed. Nobody takes care of him. His wife is out running around. She's been out all night. Before I went to work on the night shift at 11 o'clock I put him in bed. He probably fell out of bed again. He messed himself up. There's nobody to take care of him and I want action." I said "Okay. You'll get action."

So I called a caseworker and told him to meet me in front of the courthouse. In about ten minutes he was there and we walked into the house. This neighbor who had reported it came in. And of course you can't admit a person unless they agree to it. If they say, "I don't want to go in that institution," you don't admit him unless you get a court order. So we went in and you could hardly stand it in the room, the odor was so bad. We talked to this gentleman. We asked him if he would like to go to our nursing facilities. He agreed that he did. He looked as though he hadn't had a bath or maybe cleaned up for a week.

While we were there ready to return his wife came in. The first thing she was interested in, of course, was what will become of his Social security check. and I said, "Lady, you don't even worry about that. That'll be all taken care of. I'll take care of that very nicely."

Before you admit them to the home we always run them through the hospital for a check-up so that we don't carry any diseases into our home. So we called the ambulance and arranged to get him out of there that day. About 12:30 I got a call that the house was locked and the ambulance people couldn't get in. So I immediately called the caseworker. He called the sheriff and I said, "We'll go in." So we get to the home and sure enough the door was locked. But I'm pretty tall and I was able to get the screen off the window and open the window. About three fellows gave me a boost and I went in the window and got the door unlocked. We proceeded to get some clean clothing out. I couldn't stand it in the room. But one of the caseworkers proceeded to try to get some clean clothing out, and I asked if he wanted his television set. He did. He had a portable and we took that with us.

Of course his wife came back just about the time all this was going on. Again she was concerned about the check. She wasn't concerned about anything else. I think she was an alcoholic. And a finer man never walked in a pair of shoes than this man. Again I was in a position to know him. That's the reason I say in your local communities you know the people. You know how they act and you know how to take care of them.

So he was in the county home for I don't know how long. Of course then he passed away. But you wouldn't know it was the same man a week after he was in the home. He got good food and everything. He was taken care of. It's surprising the cases that we have.

We had a case of a young fellow who was a mute and a retarded girl that were in Centre Crest. They were young people. They had no right to be there. But there was no place to put them. They had no home. There was no place, and of course they were put into a nursing home. So they got to be pretty chummy, and the first thing you know they got mixed up in sex, the two of them, in the nursing home, and of course the complaints started to fly about this going on in the nursing home. So the caseworker advised us we ought to let them get married. "I think you should let them get married. I think they'd both be very happy married. I think they'd get along married," the caseworker said.

They couldn't get married of course because they weren't both of sound mind. The Registrar of Wills wouldn't bend the rules. As I said before, you have to bend the rules. And of course he wouldn't give them a license. But the caseworker never gave up. And I don't know to this day how he got them married. But they're supposedly married. He got them a home, a place to live. He got them on public assistance, got them a job working at Skills—a sheltered workshop where retarded people are taught simple and useful work—to earn some money. They're happily married.

Here's another case. This very young man is a great artist. He can paint anything he sees. He painted beautiful pictures of some of the beautiful old homes and the courthouse—in Bellefonte—any historical thing he could paint. So then he would take these pictures and try to sell them to get a little extra money. Well, of course, when you're on public assistance if you get an extra dollar you're supposed to report it. Here was a guy that was really in need. We bought several paintings off him. The judge wanted several of them for his chambers. So we get another caseworker who is from the public assistance department, and he comes in and sees these pictures. What does he do? He reports to the state that this guy is selling these pictures. Maybe he collected $100 in total out of all of them because we bought them for $20 without a frame and had them framed. And they were dirt cheap at $20. They'd be cheap at $50 or $100 as far as I am concerned. To help somebody out that was really in need for a few extra bucks.

He reports it. The first thing we knew, they were going to take his public assistance away from him and also he'd have to pay this money back. Now the commissioners had no right to get involved in this at all because it wasn't their problem. It was a problem between the public assistance department and the individual. But we got involved pretty quick, and I said we'd have somebody at the hearing on this one. We sent somebody to the hearing and after the hearing was over the man that comes up from Harrisburg to conduct the hearing said, "If I'd known it was anything like this, I'd never even have come near this case. If he just pays a dollar a year or something, just so there's something paid, we'll say he was inside the rules."

Again, I try to stress the importance of using judgment. The institutionalized couple I mentioned earlier gets along very nicely. And they've cost this county thousands and thousands of dollars before we got them married because they were always in trouble one way or another. The painter now gets along fine, causes no one any trouble, and doesn't cost the county much money. I am a great believer that we have to stay at home: knowing people, knowing their needs, and being dedicated and working hard. I had a fellow commissioner say to me, "How do you get away talking to people that way, really chewing them out in plain words?" I said, "The secret to that is knowing who you're talking to." It's that simple. If you know who you're talking to, you can stand the fire and you can fire back. But there are some people you don't know, and you've got to be very careful of how you handle the situation, because it can be delicate.

There are some sad problems to handle. You would be surprised the people that come in and get their parents' home signed over to them. They say, "Now we'll make a home for Mom or Dad for the rest of their days." We had a case where an ill man came in to see me. I didn't know him. I knew his parents—hard-working, raised a big family. He said, "How about getting mother in your Centre Crest?" I said, "You'll have to make application. That's the procedure."

So they made application, and I referred them to a caseworker. The caseworker came back and said to me, "You know the problem there is that they're living with his mother in her home. She and the daughter-in-law don't get along. And the mother's a nervous wreck. They had her to Hollidaysburg State Hospital for some treatment." I said, "Well, if you can do anything to help them out then try."

All of a sudden we get a vacancy at Centre Crest, and the lady goes into the Home. One day the caseworker came in. I said, "Whatever you do, now get a note signed so we can enter it up against the property so that we can protect the taxpayers," and he said to me, "You know she told me she already signed that over to her son." I said "What!" He said, "She told me she signed that over to her son." So I said, "Well, just follow me for a few miinutes." So I went over to the Recorder's Office to see if there was a deed put on record. There was no deed put on record. So I said, "If she did sign it over, he's never put the deed on record so we have to go up there and slap a judgment against it for about $7,500, so we can protect the people, the taxpayers."

Two hours after we did this, the son came in and put the deed on record. So everything went along fine until one day a real estate man came in to see me and he said, "You've got a judgment against this home and I got it sold." And I said, "We want our money. That's all we want. It belongs to the county commissioners." So they sold the home, and of course we got the money.

So this son who admitted his mother to the county home came in and wanted to know what I was going to do with the money. I said, "We're going to invest it and put it in a trust fund. Every month, we take out enough for burial and expenses so that your mother won't have to worry. Then she'll pay so much a month out of this fund until it's exhausted. When it's exhausted, she lives the rest of her days without paying because she doesn't have anything."

You know how long that fellow left his mother in the county home? Less than a month. And he had his mother out of the county home and got hold of that money. Now you don't believe people like that are living, but they are. It's hard to tell whatever happened to the poor mother. I just don't know. That was the end of my dealings with them.

So some people will do anything to try to get a dollar. And I'm going to tell you that I went through life, and I'm almost 70 years old, and I come from a farm where we had plenty of patches on our pants, but we always were kept clean. My mother always said it's no disgrace to be poor. It was a disgrace to not be clean. And I came up as hard a way . s anybody's come up. I've educated myself, what little education I have. And I'm telling you that there's nothing to beat being honest and being right, because anybody who will do that to their poor parents will have no respect for *any* human being.

There's one thing I would like to leave with you. Whatever you do in life, do the best you can regardless—even if it's out here digging a ditch. It might be something you don't like, but do your best. Never shirk your responsibilities or your duties. And I will assure you that you will be successful in life. Use what you have, but use it to the fullest extent and never give up. Never, never, never.

Lewis Klebanoff, an enthusiastic and humanely committed bureaucrat, reports on the problems of trying to help people, children especially, through the ponderous processes of public services. While railing against the social and medical injustice pervading so many of our "helping" services, he continues to work inside the system to bring about change that might make institutional life worth living, and the stay as brief as possible.

Chapter 11

THE DIFFICULTIES OF DOING GOOD WITH A BUREAUCRACY: SOME EXAMPLES IN CHILDREN'S SERVICES

Lewis B. Klebanoff

Planning services for children is very difficult because there are so many children and so many services. Let me just move briefly through the organic stratum of all the kinds of risks which children run and the variety of health needs they have.

Prenatal Services

One of the *greatest* services we can offer to children is to make absolutely sure that every pregnant woman gets adequate prenatal and nutritional care. An enormous amount of later trauma, stress, and social and economic expense can be prevented with adequate prenatal care. And adequate care takes in everything from adequate nutrition for mothers to their cutting down on their smoking to getting them to see the effects of drug use on fetuses. A further threat to the infant is a new kind of venereal disease of the herpes type-2 viral strain which, unless birth is by caesarean section, causes many children to die quite early.

Prenatal care for the mother in terms of her own health, concern for the whole perinatal period, as well as assuring adequacy of the health care delivery system, are essential services to children.

Research has shown that as the birth weight of premature children weighing less than 1500 grams at birth decreases, the signs of any kind of childhood disorder later in life, like mental retardation, behavior disorder, and learning disorder increase. The more mature and totally formed the baby is, the better its chances for survival in the world.

Children do not really have adequate representation. There are a lot of separate kinds of efforts on their behalf, but so far, no one has really been able to plan for them comprehensively.

Communicable Disease Control

Beyond the problem of limiting population so that there are fewer, but healthier, babies, beyond the problem of prenatal medical care for mothers and its effective delivery, and beyond the problems of neonatal care and infant nutrition lies another whole problem area of communicable disease control.

In most states, children are required to have polio shots and other types of vaccination. At this time, in the United States, more people are dying from vaccination than from smallpox. The vaccination itself is killing or maiming more people (the total number is small) than smallpox, and increasing numbers of health professionals are suggesting that polio vaccination not be administered except in high-risk areas of the world or for people going to or returning from places where smallpox is either endemic or epidemic.

Infectious disease used to kill or leave damaged great numbers of children. Today, most people assume that infectious diseaases are licked, so they don't pay much attention to them. Nevertheless, infectious diseases still do occur. And the problem that remains today, because people are so casual about them, is the secondary infections of encephalitis, meningitis, or some other infection that goes untreated or is ignored. A frequent cause of damage to infants is streptococcal infection. A child gets a sore throat so the parent goes to the drugstore and gets some kind of lozenge that eases the pain and that smoothes the child's throat and then forgets about it. But if the child has beta-hemolytic strep, he might develop heart disease, kidney disease, or any of a number of other things. And it's important to prevent secondary infection in a child by such simple things as getting cultures on sore throats that persist.

Injustice: Social and Medical

In recent years, we have talked at length about economic and educational deficiencies and social injustice. The youngsters who suffer the most from social injustices are also those who stand the greatest risk of medical disasters, primarily because they are the poorest; their families are the least educated; they get the poorest nutrition; and they get the least amount of medical care. To get medical care, they often go to a hospital clinic and sit there for six hours before anybody sees them, no matter how much they cry or are suffering.

The assumption that these people have nothing else to do but sit around for five or six hours to wait for the imperious hierarchy to decide to see them is worthy of our outrage. This is one area where the government's going to have to get more intimately involved. They're going to see that services are available when consumers need them, not just when the purveyors of service find it convenient to purvey. And yet, how can government intervene effectively in such matters?

Many poor people are afraid of doctors and hospitals, the whole medical establishment. They'll allow their children to suffer great anguish because they themselves suffer even more from the fear of what's going to be found, from the fear of having somebody treat them or their children with indignity, or invading their bodies or telling them peremptorily to take their clothes off.

Pre- and Deinstitutionalization

A further problem is keeping children from being institutionalized. Once they are placed in an institution, the chance of getting out becomes increasingly remote because the institutions themselves *cause* so much disability.

Recently, our department took some kids from an institution to somebody's house. We had a mixed class of institution and community kids, and they had never climbed a stair, had never seen a carpet, and didn't know that the switches on the wall would turn the lights on and off because, where they came from, somebody stuck a key in a hole and jiggled it and that's what turned the lights on. These kids have been deprived of the simplest kinds of human everyday experiences.

What we need to do is help prevent the institutionalization of young children by sending teams to work with their parents. This has several positive effects. First, it reaches out a hand to parents. As much as you've read about retardation, developmental disability, and cerebral palsy, nobody really cares enough to know anything about it until it happens to them. They don't really believe it. They dont't really pay attention to it. And then they think they're all alone, that it's never happened to anybody else.

Another advantage of having teams like this is that you offer parents a helping hand before the doctors, the grandparents, and other people have a chance to suggest putting the kids in an institution and to forget that they existed.

In Massachusetts, the mental health system won't take infants in our institutions anymore. They don't belong there, and we can't care for them. We will, however, offer their parents help. Some kids do need day-to-day nursing care and do have to be in some kind of a special unit. But most of them, even quite disabled, can be handled at home if their parents have skills, have a feeling that somebody knows and cares, that somebody's going to come around and visit regularly, and that there's a number they can call when they're in trouble. We teach the parents skills. The mother can show the other members of the family, for example, "This is what you do to stimulate feeding for a child who can't swallow."

Our responsibility in our agency is to care for these very disabled kids, not the generic problem of all kids. For that, nursery schools are great, and the kinds of intervention they offer and the earliest kinds of programs they provide for most kids are probably the best social investment we can have.

Day Care and Funding Faddism

I am convinced that we need day care programs and will continue to need them. But what we tend not to do in government is invest money in finding out how to do something right. One of the real problems you run into in government is that each thing has its day in the sun. For this year and maybe next, in our state, mental retardation is *in*. One of the things we too often forget is that society does not operate on logical plans. If you think that universities will create super planners who will come up with brilliant plans and then that society will adopt them because they make sense, because the plans can be shown in beautiful order on charts and graphs, and can be proved more effective and more beneficial than the existing muddle, and that political decisions are based on this, then you're dead wrong. Planners can make an input into our society, but the random ways political decisions are made boggle the mind. Yet that's reality, and it's something you've just got to learn.

The truth, of course, is that we don't know enough about day care. We've got the examples from the Israeli kibbutzim and from Russia. But those are different cultures. What about in our culture? And what about the subcultures of our culture? What do people actually do? Lots of people leave their kids with other people. Some people leave their kids locked up at home alone, and obviously, that's terrible. Do they get balanced meals? What about the dangers of fire and accidents? The need to do something about the working mother or the mother who just can't cope is obvious, and I don't deny that need. But what we tend to do in this country is go through the anguishing and very difficult process of getting the data, getting the information on which to make the wise decisions and make the multiple decisions, and then watch it all go up in smoke because the day care needed in one kind of neighborhood for one kind of ethnic group is different from another neighborhood and another ethnic group and the averaged-out government solution fits neither group.

You can set up a standardized day care system for a group of Mexican kids that just came over the border from Mexico and serve them white Protestant middle-class foods, and the kids will not eat it. We've got to have the multiplicity of response to the various subcultural needs. But *that* we don't seem to get when it comes down to legislation.

What we *do* get is some pious pronouncements and a lot of money to spend under local control. My experience is that, the quality of public servant, on the average, is higher at the federal level than at the state level, and certainly higher than at the city level, although there are marked exceptions in exactly the opposite direction. There are some brilliant people in the city government and state government, but, in general, the corruption level is the highest at the local level. So local control can, and often does, mean one huge patronage scheme having nothing to do with client need or staff quality.

I would hope that people who really know about child development and who have a passionate interest in it would get the pilot money to set up models of appropriate kinds of day care services before we just pitch billions of dollars into a pot to be passed out at the local level.

The notion that you can start with a huge federal program in one form and simply leave it to work or not work is nonsense. You've got to tune programs like you've got to tune a sports car. You've got to keep fiddling with it. You've got to change the timing a little and gap the spark plugs and do all sorts of things and try to make that thing work effectively.

Just as bad is the notion that you can be a programmatic professional completely divorced from management skills and knowledge and contemptuous of managers, who are seen as the evil guys that want to stop programs. Similarly, money management people think all the programmatic people shouldn't be allowed to deal with the public dollar.

The only thing that's going to improve that situation is management people learning something about programs and vice versa. Admittedly, that might be a little harder to do because managers see themselves as a generic group, cutting across all disciplines, and it would be very hard for them to choose what programmatic area they might want to learn something specific about.

As I said earlier, we cannot care for infants adequately in our institutions. And so, in Massachusetts, we've been refusing to take them. We recognize that we're leaving a festering problem in the community, but we recognize also that unless everybody is suffering equally, we'll never get together to solve it correctly. We'll only solve it in the old temporizing way, by shoving people into the state institution for the retarded.

Special Needs

There are other kinds of special needs, beyond deinstitutionalization. There is dyslexia, a term much in favor with parents who don't want to consider their kids retarded or emotionally disturbed. There are kids who have some kind of perceptual motor problem, which, though it doesn't fall clearly under the rubric of emotional disturbance, may, nonetheless, be a secondary characteristic of children who are not mentally retarded but who still have great difficulties in learning. There is a group of children who have been neglected or who have suffered because of great frustration. Nobody's known what to do with them or for them. Finally, there's a group (estimated at about 10 percent) of children in schools who are emotionally disturbed. All these children have special needs.

In looking at children or deciding about children's services, we have to consider that different subgroups have different values. For example, the Christian Science Church in Massachusetts is exempted from the inoculation laws. The children don't have to have the same illness prevention things that other children have to have.

Special Programs

There are generic kinds of social changes implicit in planning as well. I happen to think that the isolation of people by age or disability is rather bad. Some children with disabilities are now on *Sesame Street*, and also *Zoom* put a youngster with a disability on. I think it'll do more for the so-called normals than for the children with the disability. It gives the handicapped child at least somebody to identify with. In general, however, we don't let "normal" kids know that there is pain in the world, that people die. We keep them so antiseptically isolated from the realities of life that when they get older and find out that people become sick and disabled and hurt and suffer and die, it comes as a great shock.

Fortunately, more and more hospitals and medical schools and nursing schools are introducing courses now on death and dying. And universities are beginning a whole field of death and terminal behavior. But there are so many of thse things that interrelate. We're in a great cultural change that has inputs from so many sources, from so many disciplines, from so many power groups and influence groups that it's hard to know how to put it all in the proper perspective.

The Nature and Condition of Service Provision

Services for children are not going to be organized by any one agency. One reason is the present structure of agencies. More and more money is being spent on advocacy and less and less on services. And soon we're going to have more advocates and fewer servers. Somewhere there has to be a balance. Certainly advocacy is needed. Somebody has to speak up for kids because they can't speak up for themselves. But it's an enormously complex thing.

One thing that worries me about so many professionals today, including even a lot of physicians, is lack of disciplined respect for other people's special abilities in the system. That becomes a very dangerous kind of thing and one of the things that really troubles me. I think we ought to distinguish managerial programmatic jobs from direct technical professional service. We've got to see that respect for expertise does not decrease. An advocate can't help the person who needs intense direct expert services. On the other hand, many of us fulfill many roles, some of them direct service and some of them programmatic and advocacy services. It is not easy to develop clear and useful distinction among roles.

Every one of the assistant commissioners in Massachusetts and every one of our clinic directors do not have to be *medical* mental health professionals. As a psychologist, I couldn't have held my job a couple of years ago before the law was changed. Even though psychologists did most of the lobbying, we opened it up for social work and for rehabilitation, and for other professional fields as well. And we've got legislation pending now to open our top administrative jobs to people with master's degrees. That's a little tougher because the legislature even now wants to pay nonmedical people less than medical people. Some of the legislators cannot understand this. How can you be a doctor and not have gone to medical school? And it's even more difficult for people at the master's degree level. Answering these questions is going to be even harder, but we're trying. With luck, maybe it'll be different in the future.

Any Governor's office is in a vortex of competing and conflicting forces, and not at the top of a power hierarchy when it comes to planning and managing human services. How can next year's budget be planned when this year's has not yet been appropriated? How to plan for a reasonably steady improvement in a big program when one legislative house passes a bill to add $15 million to it and the other a bill to permanently cut the tax base for it? Terry Dellmuth, resident in that vortex, tells clearly and candidly· the many constraints—federal, legislative, professional, consumer—that must be understood and coped with in the process of trying to use the position of the Governor's office to improve human services. One piece of advice that clearly came through: to be a good planner at the state level, one has got to know the entire political process at every level of government. A tall order, but clearly presented.

Chapter 12

THE POLITICS AND ECONOMICS OF HUMAN SERVICES AS SEEN FROM A GOVERNOR'S OFFICE

Terry Dellmuth

I've been asked to give you my perspective on the economic and political factors of human service planning as seen from the Governor's office. Planning means a lot of things to a lot of people. it's obvious that in the Governor's office we don't do pure research in the human service field: we rely on the departments, professional groups, and others that we have affiliations with to give us direction. Every day we get involved in decisions that dramatically affect the delivery system. Perhaps the best way to begin is to describe just what the human service component of the Governor's Office is, and what it evolved from.

Organizing for Human Services in Pennsylvania

About 10 years ago, Governor Scranton established a Council on Human Services to open up communications between the human service agencies and state government. This Council was first located in the Welfare Department, and it was chaired by the Secretary of Welfare, a close confidante of the Governor's. This identity with the Governor was a critical factor in the successful beginning of the Council, which, after several years, was relocated to the Governor's Office of Administration and chaired by the Secretary of Adminstration.

Through the preceding administration, the Shafer years, the Council was fortunate enough to keep its continuity and its tenuous hold on permanency through the ability of its executive director, who resigned about one year before we came into office, about three years ago. The Council staff of three helped to keep lines of communication open, and, in addition, helped develop speeches for the Governor and initiate interdepartmental demonstration programs such as the Governor's branch offices.

When Governor Milton Shapp assumed office in 1971, we made a number of pivotal decisions which, to a great extent, determined the tenor of the human services ingredient of the Governor's Office. Let me say at this point that Governor Shapp's personal commitment to human services is the major factor which makes my office's job possible. But it also means that our office can't plan for more than four years at a time, even for its own existence.

It was apparent that a part-time human service special assistant with other responsibilities was not going to give the Governor's office that much of an impact. So we brought on board full-time special assistants in the fields of health, corrections, aging, manpower planning, affirmative action for women and minorities, drug and alcohol, and most recently, a new special assistant on Program and Community development.

The roles of each of these persons differ . But our central goal has been to take an interdepartmental focus on these problem areas, and, in effect, monitor system changes that we have decided on and those that we're seeking further directions for. We obviously don't have the capability to carry out changes ourselves. In many ways our role is one of helping implement agency-made plans or plans developed for us by others.

We ask each agency to accept several operating principles such as deinstitutionalization, locally run service programs, heavy consumer involvement in planning and operating services, integration of services, and so on. There are, of course, many other specific goals for each area we work in, but, with the exception of the integration of human services, these principles were relatively new for the agencies to operate under.

One of our first objectives was to involve our office in the state budgetary process. The state budgetary process, like the federal, most city, and perhaps even county budgetary processses, is largely controlled by a central office; in this case, the Governor's Budget Office. Those with experience in state government know the results of this arrangement. Each state agency approximately 9 or 10 months prior to the beginning of the new fiscal year submits its recommended budget for the coming year to the Governor's Budget Office. It is then massaged into the Governor's Budget Office recommendations which constitutionally must be balanced with the projected revenues in Pennsylvania. This has meant traditionally (since the budget office recommendations were generally followed by the Governor) that it was the budget office that was making the critical priority decisions on how to allocate scarce resources.

Governor Shapp has felt it imperative that his executive office in general, and our Office for Human Resources specifically, be heavily involved in the makeup and final decision making on his proposed budgets for the legislature. I can't overemphasize this single factor in terms of constraint on those interested in system changes or implementing planning in the human service area. Too many planners are content to build models for planned system changes but overlook the need for planning to achieve adequate funding to implement them, or to maintain basic human need programs such as income maintenance.

One of the pitfalls that we have tried to avoid is the pressure upon the Governor's Office to define human service planning as organizational and structural changes, especially at the state level. I'm asked over and over again my position on a combined human service department, on a separate department of aging, a mental health department, a youth authority, a mental retardation department, and so on. We feel organizational changes are important, and we're making some, but we don't think it's the important variable for improving services. Rather, we have tried to focus on the gaps in services on the delivery level and how they are delivered. Organizational changes should flow from that system that we developed, rather than the other way.

Limitations on State Planning

I've mentioned my reluctance to identify what we do as planning, because in many ways we are reacting to events and forces rather than controlling them. Some limitations on our ability to plan effectively are worth noting but are hardly surprising.

Federal Constraints

First, we operate under federal categorical programs and funding streams which set all kinds of limitations on us. While revenue sharing is an attempt to minimize these restraints, it has been such a drop in the bucket that it's had no real impact on the human service delivery system. Not only can revenue sharing funds not be used to match federal funds, but they must be appropriated by legislative bodies. A great bulk of the funds, therefore, were spent in tax-saving gestures for local governments. Also in many program areas revenue sharing policies have led to an actual decrease in the federal funds available for programs.

Constraints Imposed by the State Legislature

The state legislature also is the second potential force that to a great extent determines the human service delivery system. In addition to passing laws it more importantly approves and disapproves budgets. Pennsylvania's legislature has a notorious reputation among state legislatures in this country for its fiscal irresponsibility.

Much of my office's time is spent on legislative budget considerations. The 1973–1974 budget, which included many human service programs, has not been completely resolved. It sits dormant in a House-Senate conference committee because the opposition party demands that a tax relief bill be passed before program appropriations are approved. Eight months into the fiscal year, with no complete 1973–1974 budget, we had to deliver our proposed budget for 1974–1975. It was difficult to develop, for example, a rational day care plan with a fee scale involving low- and middle-income families when not only federal regulations were changing week by week as they have over the last year, but over half the budget to implement the program for the existing year hasn't been approved yet.

Similarly, when we have plans to institute a number of community-based programs for emotionally disturbed children or ex-hospital patients, it's difficult if not impossible to move forward on these programs and to plan your next year's budget when these funds haven't been approved.

As irrational as much of the legislative budgetary process appears under usual circumstances, it approaches being bizarre during an election year. One illustration that is especially timely is the debate in 1974 over the public assistance grant increase, While leaders of both parties in the legislature supported the Governor's request for a grant increase, the House Republican position was as follows. The house had recently passed a bill *cutting* $6 million from the state public assistance grant budget. This was at a time when the leaders were saying there should be a grant increase. Subsequently, the Republicans introduced a bill in the House appropriating an additional $15 million for a public assistance grant increase while, at the same time, they were vigorously pushing for a permanent tax relief bill that would eliminate any kind of grant increase.

The public and press do not understand the inconsistencies of these positions. And it's our responsibility to begin to hone in on them and point them out to the legislators themselves on both sides, and to the public, and try to begin to bring some pressure on a resolution in the direction that we want.

Consumer Interests

The consequences of inconsistencies and some of the resultant pressures that come to bear when an issue like this comes to a head can be quite serious. We get groups of welfare recipients who obviously are very upset, frustrated at the process and, whether it's a legislative problem or not, they're angry at us. Many of them come into my office screaming. I've been kicked by the very people I worked cooperatively with years ago. The Secretary of Public Welfare faces the very same kinds of pressures. Many of the legislators, especially the black caucus, who feel this pressure from their constituents directly, take out their frustrations on us, either because the legislative process isn't working, or because they want the Governor to resolve an issue. Many of the supportive orgaizations—the white middle-class organizations—such as Community Services of Pennsylvania, AFL-CIO, Catholic Conference, Council of Churches, League of Women Voters, that have coalesced around some sort of lobbying efforts for the grant increase, come at you in a much nicer, but a more naive way, saying, "Can't we compromise with those on the other side so we come up with something," even though a compromise may mean a repressive job program or it may mean other kinds of assistance we don't want.

And then we have our own legal services lawyers, that we helped organize, telling us we're all selling out because we haven't resolved it immediately or haven't increased the grant to 100 percent and just dared the legislature not to put the money into it. And of course we have those persons of a more conservative bent for whom the welfare issue invokes strong emotional reactions.

Constituent and consumer pressures then are a third variable which determine programs, sometimes at the expense of planned priorities. Citizen lobbies for mental health programs, for example, are much stronger than those for day care or criminal offenders and must be considered appropriately.

Bureaucratic Inertia and Lack of Data

Fourth, of course, is the various bureaucracies themselves which tend to have a built-in inertia to most changes. And fifth is the lack of similar definitions, similar data bases, and regrettably, many times the lack of data itself on which to build a rational plan.

Problems in System Change

I'd like to give you some examples now of the problems we deal with and some of the forces that act on us. Deinstitutionalization is a subject in itself, but I would like to touch on it briefly, because I think it is a process that exemplifies a lot of the problems we have in system changes.

Deinstitutionalization

In terms of remedying institutional use, we found it easier to cease operating health institutions, for example, such as Blossburg State Hospital, and Landis T.B. Hospital, than to disengage from mental health facilities or correctional facilities. Any attempt to close an institution has initially at least a number of opposing forces. One is the union of workers themselves who will be displaced and who are now carrying an increasingly powerful and organized voice in Harrisburg. Second is the community affected, which primarily reacts to the economic relocation, rather than the program limitations. Third, are the political leaders, whose usual prime interest is maintaining existing resources in the community. Sometimes they control these resources; sometimes they're just there to protect them.

It goes without saying that we also have tremendous community resistance to tearing down prison walls and not much less resistance when we talk in terms of dispersing the criminally insane, even to other state mental hospitals. Our primary objectives in this area have been (1) to develop community alternatives to institutionalization, (2) to improve treatment programs in institutions to better prepare for life in the community, and (3) to tighten in a gradual, but planned, manner the resources going into institutions.

In fact, though, we are not really in the business of shutting down institutions overnight, as some people would like to think. Some consumer groups such as the Pennsylvania Association for Retarded Children, (PARC) initially opposed our every attempt to construct even modular units at antiquated facilities for the mentally retarded such as Pennhurst or to transfer some patients to more modern mental health institutions that we are phasing down. This constituency is vocal and increasingly effective and must be involved in discussions. I might add that, as we become more involved, a lot of us in public positions have a tendency to react a little defensively or negatively or overreact to strident consumer demands, especially if we don't know the groups well. I've found the more we've gotten into dialogue, the more we've gotten into knowing how that group operates.

PARC, for example, has many differences of opinion. Last week the statewide PARC demanded that we not follow through on changing Embrieville State Hospital from mental health to mental retardation. Meanwhile, the local PARC chapter, concerned with Pennhurst's overcrowding, insists we go through with the change. I've been sitting on a demand to meet with the Governor 'til we could work out a position on that. We're not going to give in. There might be a timing difference.

I think it's also important to note that the unions of state human service employees, in addition to generally opposing the phasing down of their jobs in institutions, have become leaders of the opposition to increased county responsibilities for human service programs. We are told not only that state government has the commitment to maintain and develop needed programs and that county government has proven over and over again to be a complete failure in the human service field, but we're also told that most counties in Pennsylvania are dominated by rural conservative Republicans and therefore we are sounding a death knell for human service programs. We don't agree.

I point out, only incidentally, of course, that a move toward community control means that each state in the union is confronted by the fact that they will have to organize between 42 and 67 (whatever it comes out) bargaining units as opposed to the one bargaining unit that they have to deal with.

Nothing more dramatically symbolizes the basic political and economic interests that deinstitutionalization affects than the bill that passed the state house of representatives requiring legislature approval for any proposed action to decrease state institutional services. We will have fun trying to duck that one over in the Senate for the next couple of months.

We have to strive constantly to involve the various interested parties, not only to ease the initial shock of such changes, but so we become more aware of the real problems that these various groups are confronted with due to these proposed actions. This process, perhaps more than any other in my experience in state government, has brought home to me the great importance of skillful implementation of the best-laid plans. Such implementation must be based on sophisticated knowledge of, and direct communication with, all the affected forces.

Deinstitutionalization in addition to being humanitarian is economical. The taxpayers in the state are not happy with vast new investments in the human service system. Much of the additional resources we need for programs must come from an intensive planning effort and a reestablishment of priorities. This means among other things reallocating higher per-unit cost institutional programs to lower-cost community-based programs.

Consumerism

I think it worth elaborating a bit on another of our operational principles, that of consumerism. In many ways, it deals more directly with the issue of power, or more appropriately, the real location of power. Our requirement that this principle be applied to all programming efforts results in more, for example, than public assistance clients merely being put on county boards of assistance, or prisoners' or patient rights being extended. It leads to important personnel decisions: who's put in policy-level jobs, how policy decisions are arrived at, and how consumer groups are encouraged, rather than discouraged, by the state.

One reason for the basic categorical system that we now have, we think, is the result of the strong lobbying efforts of certain specific special-interest groups. But in many problem areas there's not a natural constituency that arises. Sometimes it has to be indirectly stimulated by the state. At the same time, the state personnel in these situations must minimize their defensive reactions when the result is that demands of these groups come right to their own door.

For example, we have provided grants for many elderly groups, day care groups, and citizen health organizations, only to have such bodies turn around and criticize the Governor, Secretary, or whomever for the very services that we are working together towards producing. We have to be constantly attuned also to the growing influence of, for example, a senior citizen constituency in making a policy decision. It's easier, for example, to increase the reimbursement rate for medical assistance to nursing homes when there is a greater public awareness and a pressure on us and the legislators for such increases. Our effort in these situations is one of making a specific goal, judging the potential political, public relations, consumer and economic climate, and if it seems ripe, developing an implementation plan to help bring this support to a focus.

The human service planner who gives a high priority to consumer involvement must also truly believe that the resulting, more inefficient process will also lead to constructive and meaningful programmatic recommendations and, in many cases, a more solid foundation for a permanent program.

One of the most interesting programs of consumer involvement and one of the highest priority ones that we had early in the administration has been the Governor's Action Center. This center, now manned by over 30 employees in the Governor's office receive toll-free telephone calls from citizens throughout the state with problems that are relevant to the state government. Much more than an information and referral center, it gives a disgruntled citizen a chance to have an immediate fair hearing so to speak and to appeal a decision or a lack of decision by state agencies with which they have disagreed. The Governor has made it clear to his Cabinet that he expects immediate action or immediate attention given to these complaints.

I don't mean to suggest that every citizen is satisfied after their call, and indeed we haven't even extended into the Philadelphia area yet. But there are at least a couple of relevant results of this program for human service planners in addition to the consumer involvement aspect itself.

First, it is a program that is available to all citizens regardless of incomes, age, sex, or race. There's no biased constituency. It's not an urban-based program, nor a program that anybody can say "Hey, it's for somebody else." It should, we hope, have a broad-based support and therefore, become permanent.

Second, by keeping records of the problems called in and the solutions or lack of solutions provided, we are given an unsolicited and instantaneous review of many of the state programs that either are mired in bureaucracies or perhaps don't exist when they need to. Sometimes this has even led to disagreements with policies of the state agency or state agency head. In these cases, this results in the Governor's personal intervention with a cabinet member.

Perhaps this is the best point to put in my usual plug for human service planners and providers to become thoroughly knowledgeable and involved in the political process itself. The political system as structured is still potentially a very democratic system; how it's operated has led to its problems. At the very least it offers us all a better knowledge of the pressure points, the change points, to help us implement those things we're working on. The quality of elected officials, while far from ideal, is still rising. State legislators today are increasingly independent and more representative of the electorate. The increase in numbers of black state legislators, for example, has led to an organized black caucus which in the past 2 years has been instrumental in pushing forward some of the human service programs.

The less an elected official has to be beholden either to a political party or to monied interests, the more likely he or she is to be receptive to programs for people in need and not vote on the basis of a party rule or a caucus rule, such as that still operating in the House of Representatives in one party. In that situation, one is told which way to vote; and it still happens. We had about 28 newly elected representatives this past election, the highest percentage of turnover. There was great hope that the unit rule would break, that there'd be some independence provided by the opposition party. (I'm biased of course, Take with a grain of salt what I'm saying.) There were some excellent candidates elected, 25 to 35 years was the average age. Within a month, however, they were in the old mold and voting with the party on all the critical bills right down the line.

Civil servants are becoming more politically active, and within limits this is to the good. Today, especially at the federal level, and increasingly in the Commonwealth, some elected legislators have emerged as knowledgable advocates for improved human services. Their increased involvement in our planning efforts is essential.

The Legal System as a Planning Tool

One of the most useful, but still underutilized instruments for social systems planners are the courts and the legal system. Not only does the legal system offer consumer protection tools, but it is an arsenal that can be used to help implement planning goals. For example, the Pennsylvania Right to Treatment Agreement guaranteeing public education for mentally retarded children from ages 3 to 21 was something that was developed before Governor Shapp took office. Once the suit was filed and his staff was in office, we negotiated a settlement that in effect broadened the purpose of the original suit. Such a settlement is costly and was initially opposed within the administration by key officials. But with the support of the Governor, we accomplished a settlement that already has had a tremendous impact on education and treatment programs. While there's a long way to go for the mentally retarded, it has suggested some directions for some of the other areas on the horizon.

Similarly, the Governor has proposed additional funds in each of his budget proposals to begin to eliminate the system of peonage in our mental institutions. These funds have been eliminated each year by the legislature as a nonpriority item. For that reason, we have looked favorably, although unofficially, on various lawsuits that have been brought against the state peonage system. Sometimes substantial program changes, especially those costing substantial funds, are just not possible to pull off within the existing legislative and administrative budgetary process. And the court system can be a tremendous help in these situations.

I caution, however, against an overreliance on the court system, because many settlements that are worked out and more frequently. ordered by the courts are superficial and perhaps even repressive or negative in the directions that we are working towards.

Coordination of Health Services

Turning to the field of health for just a moment, our perception of the health system has been that it probably more than any other human service system has been dominated by the providers. So that, obviously, a good deal of our effort has been to, in effect, encourage the development of counterbalances to this. I think that forces are at work on their own to produce some of that counterbalance.

One reason for creating a position in our office to coordinate health services has been the proliferation of health services among several state agencies. The majority of state health services were originally located in the welfare department because of the basic distrust by legislators and governors of health providers, and the heavy influence that they would have on a health department run strictly by health professionals. It is our feeling that as these influences are becoming counterbalanced that we should make attempts to further strengthen the health department role in overall health planning and operation while making sure that health decisions are made in the context of the whole human service delivery system.

There's no question that our greatest health pressure still comes from organized doctors, hospitals, nursing home operators, pharmacists, and so on. But these groups are becoming increasingly constructive in their goals because the public pressure demands that they not just be seen as professional lobbies out of the Dark Ages. But they are competing with other growing influences with different points of view. And as this still basically privately financed system becomes more publicly financed, this influence will wane even further.

State or Local Control

For many years, those involved in human service planning in Pennsylvania at the state level have been evenly split between those favoring a state-administered system and those favoring local or county systems. Tragically, decisions in this regard were made within individual programs which led to the programmatic schizophrenia in today's system. We've commissioned a number of reports inside and outside of government to evaluate options and to get the bureaucrats and others evaluating, thinking ahead, thinking of where the system change is going to go, and working together towards them. And I should add that consumer groups are involved in it. Nobody agrees entirely, and we find that a lot of the consumer groups now by working together on planned changes are beginning to have less resistance to things that they opposed initially, but they understand it better and want to focus on what they want, rather than on what they're opposed to.

In addition to the consumer organizations that have been involved and the unions of state employees, that have expressed considerable opposition to this goal, we have an additional critical problem to address in this regard: the role of county government itself in assuming more leadership and involving a meaningful and interrelated delivery system. There are a lot of new things on the horizon that we have already started to implement and that will affect the delivery system in the counties, such as the Older Americans Act, even the movement of economic development councils into human service planning. This cannot be done overnight. We cannot have economic planners really making the basic decisions for us right away. But these are all to the good. And I think that those involved in county-level planning efforts will probably be where the action is.

The Future of State Planning and Planners

Where are we going? What can we expect to be different? Why do we expect human services to be more effective in the future than they are now? In dealing with problems like these, those of us working in the system incline to be optimistic; we're certainly not objective. We're in the battle day in and day out. I probably ought to pose the question to you on the outside who are looking at the system more objectively and say, "What are we doing wrong? What could we do better from your perspective?" and then tell you what some of the restraints are. I think we're optimistic. We feel that some changes aren't as visible as they might be, but that the directions we are going are good, and we're building good foundations. So we're optimistic, and a lot of that I've tried to paint here.

Although we've moved into regionalization in trying to decentralize operations, some goals have yet to be arrived at. I've come to the conclusion, and we've certainly been operating on this, that we've got to draw in a lot of outside people, not what I call model-builders per se, but concerned laypeople who are thinking realistically of the problems we struggle with.

Restraints on Future Planning

In closing, I would like to try to outline a number of restraints to effective future operations. First of all, there is the state system itself: 115,000 employees, 70 percent civil service, the other 30 percent patronage controlled essentially by county chairmen or state legislators.

Secondly, our personnel system is a scattered system. This is one of the things I've been working on and feeling very frustrated about, because we need legislation for a central personnel system. We have a personnel office for the patronage jobs, and in the Office of Administration which deals with classification of jobs; we have a civil service system. We need, in my opinion, a central personnel office with all those separate offices merged. We need a development of a career ladder system that enables anybody to move from one level to another and that deemphasizes educational requirements as a prerequisite for employment in certain jobs.

Third, we need the legislative and political processes. The Governor constantly uses the analogy of the legislature as a Board of Directors. His biggest shock in state government was coming into a situation where at least half the board of directors are working against you. If you're going to be working as a Governor or in the Governor's Office, you have accepted the fact that you're going to have to be a political animal.

Another aspect is the administration of state government agencies; to what degree does an administrator run them, and to what degree do they run themselves? That's a decision that any chief executive has to face and make some decisions on. Some just get completely lost and go off and do their own bit. Others, like the present Governor of Pennsylvania like to get involved in all kinds of decisions, and obviously, one should participate in decisions with the cabinet officers. Nevertheless, a lot of the critical decision making is made right in the departments. There's no point in fooling ourselves that way. Some people do.

Restraints on Future Planners

How, you may ask, does one thrive in such an atmosphere? What will the future planner need to work effectively? I think perhaps I learned my survival skills from participation a few years ago with radical groups, where the emphasis was placed on building a solid philosophical goal and communion among people with that goal. Now there are a lot of people in the top levels of government who only make the decision. There are too many people around who don't care what is being decided or who don't work towards anything. So in one aspect it's important for us to know what we want to do in each job that we get into, not in order to have the answers when we go into it, but to have the philosophy of how we want to operate so that when we become the focus of disenchantment for all kinds of people, we do know what to do and can get all kinds of help from people. That's one area of support that for me is essential. When you're really asking what is worthwhile, you have to know what to measure the things you're doing against, and other people help you measure that.

These are personal restraints. One of the great fears I have (and a lot of us in a similar position have it) is not recognizing when to get out. When do you need a sabbatical? When do you need to just get out because you're becoming ineffective? Unless you have a reference group, you grow out of touch.

I think a family, just your own personal life, is important too. We have people going through all kinds of traumatic personal life experiences and falling apart on the job because it's tough to maintain or go into the kind of pressures these jobs entail when you don't have at least a fairly stable personal life. It's important to judge what you want to be doing personally during the period of time that you're going to stay in the public limelight.

Because of the emphasis placed upon individualism by most Americans, according to Dr. Frederick R. Eisele, there is a strange and inevitable logic which leads to the ironies of categorical programs as the means our Federal government uses to meet human needs. Categorical programs are seen as a compromise between more extensive planning and individualism. Special interest groups generate the political pressure needed to promote the required legislation. The legislation has to be politically saleable so the target population has to be specified, and be deemed worthy of help. It is the specification of target population and authority which inexorably leads to fragmentation of service delivery on the local level. But the final piece of irony is in the 1973 Federal legislation which created yet another categorical program which was implemented in the form of local services planning and coordinating authorities targeted specifically on the elderly: Area Agencies on Aging (AAA). The very specification of the target population (i.e., 60 years of age or older) creates an artificial class of highly heterogeneous individuals which makes effective programming almost impossible. Yet there is no doubt that the controversies generated both in the academic arena and on the local and state level will insure the inclusion of the elderly in whatever social planning is done on the state and federal level.

Chapter 13

ADMINISTERING SERVICES BY AGE CATEGORY: THE ELDERLY

Frederick R. Eisele

Any discussion of administration of services for the elderly needs to begin with an understanding of how categorical services emerged historically. Only then can services by age category, and services to the elderly in particular, be seen in their proper context. Within the limits of time and space, I will outline this development, say something about the impact of such thought and action on planning, and finally speculate about the future of services to the aged.

Historical Development of Categorical Services

The story of how social services emerged for specific groups in need can best be told from a political perspective. The prevailing ethic of individualism dictated that personal needs were the concern of the individual (i.e., because the problem was generated by the person, it logically had to be solved by the person), or by his or her family, or at most, by their physician or minister. As these private resources became inadequate to growing needs for services in a rapidly industrializing society, the ethic required that the needs of the mentally retarded, the ill, dependent children, the elderly, etc. be redefined as *special cases*, as exceptions to a rule which said that if you were "normal," you wouldn't need assistance or support.

Politically, this "requirement" was turned into a convenient strategy. As it turned out, it was easier to mobilize constituent support for and attract legislative attention to these special cases than for broad, ill-defined needs. For example, on the one hand, friends and supporters of retarded children could be identified, rallied and counted on for volunteers in a nationwide fund-raising campaign; on the other hand, state and federal legislators on relevant committees could be buttonholed, lobbied, and influenced on specific bills which they knew carried organized voter support. Ultimately, mobilizing political support for persons with special categories of needs had to take the form of an interest group, much like the antisaloon league of the 1930s, or General Motors, or Nader's consumer research groups of today.

Two outcomes of this political development should be noted in passing. Although they were probably not intended benefits, the emergence of interest groups and subsequent legislation for particular categories of needy persons produced a growing number of experts, both political and academic, who generated the beginnings of a knowledge base about this population. Moreover, planning and future development of services for such categories or groups became focused, and therefore more controllable, by virtue of their specificity. In the long run, however, as we've begun to see in the 1970s, there are unintended costs as well, such as fragmentation and duplication of services. This fragmentation was true for the poor and disabled, as well as for age categories, as is evident from the fact that poverty, disability, and age are in no way exclusive categories.

Services by Age Group

All societies recognize changes in abilities across the life span and accordingly assign different rights and duties by age. In modern, industrial societies, chronological age has taken on an exaggerated importance as a convenient and apparently equitable standard of eligibility for an array of rights and duties. Most states set, for example, an age eligibility level between two and three years for entry into preschool, sixteen years for an automobile license, and minimum ages for marriage licenses, while the federal government has age eligibility levels for registration for military service, voting, holding public office, retirement, and claiming social security benefits. Thus, age has long been used as a legal category qualifying rights and duties, including rights to social services.

Historically, social services categorized by age first developed for children and youth, and only later for the aged. This sequence does not necessarily reveal a value priority on children as much as it does the historically unpredicted and still growing percentage of elderly which appeared rather rapidly in the twentieth century. (The proportion of the population over 65 years of age rose from 3 percent in 1900 to almost 10 percent in 1970.) Children and youth emerged as a category with increasing distinction in the late nineteenth century because of the impact of industrialization on child labor and because of widely supported movement for compulsory public education. It is worth noting that education itself can be properly considered a social service. Yet, the generally favorable public attitude toward education contrasts sharply with the usually questioning and reluctant public attitude toward publicly supported personal or family social services.

The Children's Bureau, emerging in the Department of Health, Education and Welfare in the early decades of this century, and the struggle for a separate juvenile court system were parts of a movement to achieve justice for a category that was clearly at a disadvantage by virtue of age. Public recognition of the elderly as a disadvantaged or somehow unequal category came more slowly.

One can trace the gradual emergence of public concern for older Americans in three distinct policy stages, which correspond to the policy sectors of income maintenance, health insurance, and social services, over a period of 40 years. Although there had been a social insurance movement prior to World War I, only the devastating effect of the Great Depression on the elderly was sufficient to provoke a federal response of setting a universal income floor for retired workers, which was the 1935 Social Security Act. This initial effort was well behind most European nations, where income maintenance programs dated to Bismarck's state pension plan of the 1800s.

The struggle between the proponents of health insurance and its major opponent, the American Medical Association, went on for years before a medical insurance bill, confined to those over 65, was finally passed in the form of Medicare in 1965. Thus, there was a hiatus of almost a quarter century before public concern was again aroused over the elderly, this time as a part of the Kennedy-Johnson antipoverty programs of the mid-1960s. Yet, in the 1950s and early 1960s significant changes had been occurring, despite the absence of concrete legislation. The U.S. Senate formed a Special Committee on Aging, and this group remains today one of the best sources of information about public policy. The interest groups alluded to above were also beginning to emerge, formed by and on behalf of the elderly. The National Retired Teachers Association allied with the American Association of Retired Persons to form a larger more powerful organization, and the National Council for Senior Citizens, a labor-oriented group, appeared in the early 1960s to mobilize support for Medicare. There were other groups as well. One was the Gerontological Society, an association dedicated to research on aging, which began to develop a knowledge base on older populations in both biological and social sciences, and recently in policy-related research. It began in the 1940s.

In the same year that Medicare passed as Title 18 of the Social Security Act, Congress passed an Older Americans Act. While not provided with much funding in its early years, it did establish an Administration on Aging with HEW, and this organization grew to have a central role in national policy for the elderly.

So by 1970, the two basic problems of older citizens—loss of income and loss of health—had been met by public programs in at least a rudimentary way. What needed implementation was the concept of social services to complement income maintenance and, in the instance of health, to postpone or even obviate the need for costly institutionalization. Pressure for some systematic, national program or services to the elderly was built up in the late 1960s and early 1970s. The second (decennial) White House Conference on Aging in 1971 focused the issues more sharply but it was 1973 before the "Comprehensive Services Amendments" were signed into law, widely referred to as the "new" Older Americans Act.

The Area Agencies on Aging

The most important piece of this new Older Americans Act in regard to services administration was Title III, which created authorities for planning and coordinating services to older residents in every state. These *Area Agencies on Aging*, (AAA) as they came to be known, functioned to plan and to centralize services for older agencies. The Area Agencies were funded for three years, during which time most were able to open their doors, and were renewed in 1976 for another three years. After 1979, it is widely assumed that their costs are to be absorbed by localities—states or counties.

The major problems of these new entities were typical of organizations in early stages of development: staffing, responding to state office directives, and fulfilling annual plan requirements. Problems of agencies in rural areas differed sharply from those in cities. Rural agencies found reluctance to utilize public services: in part, because support networks of family, friends, and church were still strong; in part, because even such access services as information and referral or transportation were perceived as tainted with a welfare stigma. Urban agencies, on the other hand, commonly found no reluctance toward use of services, but rather a different set of problems altogether. One of the most severe was that of turf guarding—well-established agencies with track records or partial involvement with the elderly regarded the AAA's as upstarts who threatened to reduce the size of their own hard-fought-for slice of federal or state funds, as well as to take away some of their own constituents.

By mid-1976 some Area Agencies had made an important difference in the provision of services to the elderly in their jurisdictions, while others had not yet seriously gotten off the ground. The performance of most was mixed, and most AAA directors would probably caution with the familiar "it's too early to tell."

Title XX

An even more important piece of legislation from a Social Services perspective is Title XX of the Social Security Act (1975). This is an omnibus social services bill with the major goal of reducing dependency, particularly among children, the handicapped, and the elderly. Potentially, Title XX funds are an enormous resource for Area Agencies to draw on. The citizen participation requirement, also, gives a voice to providers and consumers that was not formalized before. Eligibility requirements, however, have restricted the use of these funds to low-income individuals and families. Difficulties have arisen because of the fact that there is a sizeable percentage of elderly just above the required income level, and because the costs of administering the income (means) test have been disproportionately high. In mid-1976, implementation of Title XX was still undergoing significant modifications, although it remained the major source of social service funding for older Americans.

Impact of Age Categorical Services

No one yet knows what long-run effect the Area Agencies will have on the administration of services to the elderly, but few doubt that they have aroused public awareness of service needs far beyond what it had been. One example is chore services for older home owners no longer able to take down storm windows, clean gutters, etc. This mundane instance of a typical social service can only be appreciated when it is realized that a main reason for older persons leaving their home of many years is their inability to cope with maintenance chores, and that relocation—to the home of an adult child or a group home—is terribly disorienting and is usually the first step toward dependence and institutionalization, all of which are infinitely more costly than staying in one's own home.

There is a larger question raised by the new social services strategy embodied in the Area Agencies, and this is whether such an age-categorical program might not be draining off needed resources from other categorical groups. Such a concern, of course, is the traditional double-edged sword of any group-specific program: while identifying needs and resources, it also overidentifies the group in question. This use is not confined to the social services sector and, in fact, threatens to emerge more sharply in the income maintenance programs, where increasing payroll tax bites for all wage earners could generate a resentful backlash against the elderly in the future.

Another outcome is possible, however; a successful services strategy via Area Agencies could serve as a model for all age groups, which happened in 1965 with Medicare. Although not widely known, Medicare was in a sense a compromise on national health insurance. Instead of health insurance for all, the compromise came in the form of an experiment with a "deserving" sector of the population—those over 65. If national health becomes a reality, it will most likely draw heavily on the Medicare experience, which has been successful for the most part. After a decade, there should be enough evidence to evaluate the effectiveness of the Area Agencies; but it would be a surprise if the country were ready for a national, noncategorical program of social services by that time.

The Future of Social Services

The development of social services in general, and of social services for the elderly in particular, will take many directions in the next 5 to 10 years, if for no other reason than that the 50 states already have taken different approaches in their various programs. Some states have only a few Area Agencies, while Pennsylvania, for example, has 47. The larger changes, however, are as likely to be affected by shifts in the boundaries of age categories as they are by administrative developments.

An inkling of the undercurrents of change can be seen in some paradoxical trends. There are signs of both a growing age-consciousness among older citizens, for example, as well as a simultaneous move toward age-irrevelant categories for older populations. Age-consciousness has been increased simply by the amount of age-specific legislation generated in the past decade, and also the citizen participation requirements written into some of that legislation. Thus, state plans for services for the elderly are required to be aired in advance in statewide hearings. The Area Agencies have their own citizen advisory boards, some of which are becoming more vocal as they learn the game.

In the future, say the next 30 to 50 years, the age-consciousness of older citizens may well be even more pronounced as better educated cohorts move into the age status of elderly. The generation of elderly in the 1940s and 1950s, far less educated than its children or grandchildren, was largely quiescent in politics. Each new cohort arrives with slightly more schooling than its predecessor, and it is widely known that education is a prime predictor of political awareness and participation. Future, more politicized generations of elderly, looking out for their own interests, may well organize further and focus particularly on the remaining policy sector—social services—which links and complements the first two policy sectors of income maintenance and health care.

On the other hand, age categories may become much less relevant to social services in the future. One indicator is the criticism recently launched against the retirement age of 65. Set during the Depression, when life expectancy was shorter and there was a need to make room in the labor force for unemployed younger workers, the age of 65 has been seen as both discriminatory (for racial minorities with lower life expectancies) and arbitrary (for both those occupations wishing to retire earlier and those seeking to prolong their work lives).

Economists and other have for some time noted the lack of empirical basis for the 65 eligibility level for social security and for most compulsory retirement regulations. Early retirement options in the auto and steel industries, available for over a decade now, mean that an increasing percentage of the blue-collar labor force is withdrawing in their mid 50s, with an average of 20 years of life remaining. The Department of Labor has long noted the mobility problems of workers over 45, and in fact takes that age as its definition of "older worker."

Bernice Neugarten, a University of Chicago social psychologist, has recently called attention to the increasing irrelevance of age 65 by using the terms "Young-Old" (55 to 75) years and the "Old-Old" (75 plus years) to distinguish those persons who have retired around 55, are relatively secure financially, and are in relatively good health,from those persons 75 plus who are beginning to run into serious chronic illness problems, are losing friends and spouses, and with it the physical mobility required for social independence. Even more recently, the Federal Council on Aging has called for research on the "frail elderly," those over 75, (mostly women, because of the lower male life expectancy) who run increasing risks of greater dependency and institutionalization.

What these recent efforts at redefinition imply beyond the growing irrelevance of the traditional age 65 is the great heterogeneity of older persons, and consequently, the range of their social service needs. There has been a tendency, stemming from the aura surrounding "65" to lump "the aged" into a single category, to assume homogeneity without examination. As the above criticisms should show, however, "the aged" are in fact highly differentiated. The social service needs of the unemployed school teacher of 45, the newly retired steelworker of 55, the grieving widower of 65 or the 75 year-old woman with a broken hip are needs which run the gamut of the entire range of social services.

With this greatly expanded notion of age-specific needs, age eligibility itself may become less relevant, or at least change its current structure. After all, if "aging" refers to a series of categories composed of persons 45 years old and older, one is referring to nearly half the population. And here may be seen a potential resolution of the paradox noted earlier between the apparent increase in both age-consciousness and the trend toward an age-irrelevant society. If age-consciousness sharpens among future cohorts, and does so at an earlier age in the life span, then age-specific social services, i.e., by age category may come to be seen as only a convenient guide to a *type* of service rather than as a criterion for eligibility. Ultimately we should come to a more European view of social services as a complementary policy sector for which *all* citizens may have occasional need. Under these conditions social services would be accessible on a universal basis, and "not for the the poor alone."

Summary

Administration of services to the elderly needs to be understood within the context of the political development of categorical services in general, of which age-categorical services are a special case. The political context includes both the American value of individualism, which made recognition of need for services difficult to legitimize, and the consequent strategy of seeking support for special need by means of interest or pressure groups. Interest groups on behalf of the elderly emerged gradually in the 1950s and especially, 1960s, and it was 1973 before federal legislation created local services planning and coordinating authorities targeted specifically on the elderly. These local Area Agencies on Aging have already had an important impact especially as citizen advocacy and public awareness agents. Social services to the elderly in the future will depend in part on the success of the Area Agencies, but will be much more affected by the greater education of and therefore higher probability of political involvement in future generations of older Americans.

A critical moment in the formation of federal, state and local relations was the combining of the departments of Health, Education, and of Welfare into one administrative structure by President Eisenhower. The Department of Health, Education and Welfare's record can be summarized in its development of categorical funding targeted to specific populations as the major means of dealing with human needs. The nightmare quality of this method is summarized by Dr. Anthony Broskowski on the following pages, a quality which has made the federal record in addressing human needs a basis for questioning the legitimacy of the federal government. The incredible level of complexity, duplication, and fragmentation of services requires an almost superhuman effort to comprehend. Dr. Broskowski successfully makes such an effort and presents here in a lucid fashion the problems of marshalling the diverse streams of funding into a roughly coordinated organized assault on the human service needs of metropolitan area. While the focus is on mental health programming, this focus serves only to highlight the many dimensions of, as he phrases it, the nightmare of categorical funding.

Chapter 14

THE NIGHTMARE OF CATEGORICAL FUNDING OF SERVICES: PUTTING IT TOGETHER AT THE LOCAL LEVEL

Anthony Broskowski

Intergovernmental Relations and the Public–Private Interface in Human Services

Intergovernmental relations can include the relations among federal, state, county, and other local government units, as well as the relations that exist among the executive, legislative, and judicial branches of any level of government. One could also talk about the relations among agencies at any given level, for example, between the city school system and the city parks, or between the state mental health and the state welfare, or between the Department of Health, Education and Welfare and Housing and Urban Development. All of these dimensions must also be considered along with the public–private dichotomy, which isn't really as sharp as a dichotomy as it used to be, and the future is likely to blur even further the formerly sharp distinctions between the public and the private sectors.

A friend of mine who is a political scientist told me that the classical theory of intergovernmental relations is that each level of government is supposed to have a unique responsibility. For example, national defense is supposed to be a federal responsibility; education is a local responsibility; highways should be built by the state. That approach soon proved very outmoded and there evolved a "marble-cake theory," the realization that everything would blend with everything else. All levels of government would get involved in all functions. And this approach is presently the accepted case, although it has become such a mess now that all levels of government are trying to sort out again those more rational approaches to what various levels of government should do for any given *categorical* function such as education, corrections, or welfare.

Programming Categorical Function

When I say categorical, I mean a special program for a special category of people, for example, blinded veterans from World War II. Categorical is contrasted to a noncategorical, or general purpose program that does not restrict itself by age, income, type of problem, or other eligibility or classification approaches.

Let me back into this topic with some very recent history of the 1950s and 1960s. There has been a lot of intergovernmental rivalry and pluralistic ignorance and cross-agency completion is very common. In HEW, it's likely that the people in the health section do not know what the people in education are doing. Rivalry exists because they directly compete for the same funds from Congress. Ignorance can be tolerated because each agency feels it has its own safe funding source. It may not be safe to admit you need another agency's help! *And so it is at the level of local and state government*: The parks and the school people may really be competitive rather than cooperative, because they both draw on the same mayor's budget.

There is also rivalry between levels of government. The "feds" blame the people at the state level for having inadequate bureaucrats "who can't run things." And the state people talk about the poor quality of local government. Lower levels of government criticize the insensitivities of higher levels.

In an excellent piece of satire, David Kennedy (1972) promulgated the "law of appropriateness." This law says that the level of government most appropriate to deal with a given problem is the level where one is presently employed. The first corollary of this law says that other levels of government are basically untrustworthy and require constant supervision and observation. A great deal of time and effort must therefore be expended to find out what they are up to, usually by meetings or other techniques of coordination. (He didn't mention "bugging" but that has become another popular approach.) The second corollary is that the decision about appropriateness does not include the willingness to assume the actual operational phase of the program, except at the local government level where no choice exists. They have to run it whether they want to or not. The third corollary states that duplication of effort at various levels is not wasteful and inefficient but rather is essential to the preservation of the intergovernmental system. There is also a "law on finance and taxation," that level of government most appropriate to finance a given governmental program is any level other than the one where one is presently employed. Kennedy goes on in a rather cynical and satirical fashion to document this intergovernmental rivalry and ignorance.

Historically, the federal government stayed out of the business of human services planning, funding, and delivery until the 1930s when the Depression showed that private charitable or local government programs were inadequate. Rising social mobility in the 1940s and 1950s also stimulated the federal and state governments to pick up the expensive custodial services formerly provided by close-knit extended families. Veterans from World War II also sought and received significant health and education benefits. The 1960s saw the Civil Rights Movement and the War on Poverty the ideology that only the federal government could insure adequate and equitable services to those most in need.

In the 1960s the federal government tried to define "the needs" of the citizen. Every time a new need would be identified, a new program would be started just for that need. For a variety of reasons both the executive and legislative branches of government supported this catagorical approach. It was also favored by special interest groups of service consumers and providers. Professionals like the approach because it usually promotes their own welfare and training. Administrators at all levels liked it because it gave the semblance of accountability through direct line control of funds.

Now the categorical approach seemed a reasonable thing to do at the time, because Congress assumed that state and local governments were unwilling or unable to assist the poor, the black, the sick, and other special need groups, and the federal government believed in deficit spending. Each of these newly authorized programs gradually built up a bureaucracy to administer it and a very vocal constituency to promote its continual expansion.

Unfortunately, the categorical approach has produced, over time, a set of problems. These narrow categorical programs were largely unplanned and are increasingly recognized as inefficient and ineffective in meeting the comprehensive human service needs of individual citizens. More specifically, their complexity, fragmentation, rigidity and growth is alarming. Since 1960, the number of categorical programs within HEW alone has grown from 100 to more than 300 as of 1973. Fifty-four of these overlap with each other in some way, the 36 overlap with programs in other cabinet-level administrative units of government. The average state has between 80 and 100 separate human service agencies at the state level. As of 1973 the average community had between 400 and 500 local human service agencies which are government sponsored.

Federal rules and regulations for these 300-plus HEW programs are highly prescriptive, restrictive, duplicative, and conflicting. There are 1200 pages of regulations devoted to the administration of these programs in the federal register. And for every page of regulation there are, on the average, ten pages of interpretive guidelines. All these regulations require separate bookkeeping procedures, separate accounting for each grant, duplicative and sometimes conflicting reporting requirements. State and local matching rates vary with no apparent reason from 0 to 90 percent matching. There are strict prohibitions against joint funding and combining and comingling funds for various programs. Local level service agencies couldn't financially coordinate their separate programs if they wanted to.

Furthermore, in 1969, less than half of these programs were fully appropriated and by 1971 only a third were fully funded. It is estimated that HEW's authorized service delivery programs, which cost $9 billion, would cost $250 billion if fully funded.

One example comes from social services. Title IV-A is a federal program of matching state money to deliver social services to welfare clients. This program has created all kinds of problems. HEW officials complained about the lack of control, because they initially had to put out three dollars for every one dollar the state put up, regardless of the total amount. Congress finally placed a ceiling on total spending in Title IV-A. The Congress complained because the state people asking for the money were not specific about what services they would provide. The clients complained because the funded services were unrelated to their needs. For example, the state government said, "We'll fund day care, we'll fund counselling, we'll fund family services," when they might not be the solutions to the primary problems faced by those citizens in Community X. The state planners complained about the uncertainity of the funds for long-range planning. The caseworkers and the professionals complained about being caught in the middle. Poor people complained about being caught at the bottom. All these service programs in turn became connected to the welfare program, which is attached to a stigma. Many did not want to use the services that were made available.

Categorically organized programs are also inefficient, fragmented, and very duplicative. In 1969, for example, HEW reported that 75 percent of the federal discretionary dollars available for health in a given geographical area of the United States were all going to one city in the form of seven different health grants. Each grant required a separate governing body of citizens, professionals, etc., and so seven different advisory boards and commissions, having overlapping membership and charters, existed within one city.

In another city six different day care–child development programs were all operating under separate auspices, each utilizing different federal categorical money for support. Chattanooga, Tennessee had twelve different federally funded drug abuse programs, each with its own special ties, facility, clients, information and referral, unique eligibility requirements, data processing and financial accounting and purchasing systems. Some other independent studies showed in two states that when it comes to physicians and social workers, they actually spent less than 25 percent of their time practicing medicine and counseling clients. These professionals were being grossly underutilized because they spent so much time on these duplicative kinds of support activities (i.e. those 1200 pages of regulations). These programs were inefficient and ineffective.

Viewed from the perspective of any organizational level in the system, the categorical programs appear to be chaotic. Offices in Washington cannot bring them together. Regional administrators in the ten federal regions cannot coordinate them. State governors are frequently bypasssed altogether as the money flows to local governments and such nonprofit grantees as universities or service organizations.

Very narrow eligibility requirements exist when seeking help from government-sponsored programs at the local level. "We only treat alcoholics from World War II who are also poor." Many times a program won't accept you because you live on the wrong side of a line that runs through your street. You may not even know where to get service. Or you know where the service is, you're eligible, but you can't get there because there's no transportation since it was built in the suburbs to be easily reached by the staff.

HEW did a study and found out that somewhere between 86 and 95 percent of most of its clients had a need for more than one type of service. A study found that the probability of getting accepted by the first human service agency you go to for help is about 0.4. Similarly depressing statistics have been found by others. Worse yet, the probability of a connective referral from one agency to another runs around 0.17!

From the client's perspective, an effective program must be accessible, available, and provide sufficient continuity. It is pointless to help a person with multiple problems in only one of these problems. Expert carburetor repair in a car without checking the battery brakes, and gears will be worthless because the car won't work if all the parts are minimally adequate. So it is for many citizens. Effectiveness must be viewed as a measure of the client's total level of functioning and not restricted to criteria based on narrow professional views of excellence.

There's also some evidence that the more programs that exist, the less likely it is that the clients' needs will be met. This phenomenon has a lot to do with the relative energy that goes into boundary maintenance behavior of subsystems within the general system. The more subsystems that exist, the more energy must go into keeping those boundaries maintained and developing limited linkages between them. Unfortunately, subsystems frequently find it in their own short run interests to keep their boundaries impermeable.

The fact is that the complex eligibility criteria generally serve more to select clients out of, rather than into, programs. I once developed what I call the "toilet-flushing model" to describe the intake and referral methods frequently found in classical child-guidance clinics. A waiting list is analogous to a toilet bowl. A pool of clients are stored and then as the residents, social workers, and psychology interns need a good training client, all one has to do is pull one off the list. It's like flushing the toilet. But generally all of the clients are not on the list. They can be kept on a waiting list, however, because it's useful to claim a tremendous need for more money when you go to charitable organizations each year. You get into "input-budgeting," that is, you claim to need money based on the potential input that is lined up, rather than what the output has been. It can be shown that as the limited clients get discharged. others get creamed off the list based on professional staff interests.

Does anyone deny we have a problem? Some people are still very much in favor of this categorical approach because they feel if you eliminate it there will be many groups of high-risk individuals who will get hurt or neglected if this system is not there protecting their special interests. The question is, can you develop an alternative approach to human services and intergovernmental relations that avoids these wasteful and fragmented efforts while maintaining accessible services for those clients who need them?

Alternative Approaches

One approach to solving some of the problems of categorical programs essentially involves a shift in political and financial responsibilities among federal, state, and local government. Nixon called it "New Federalism,"; Johnson previously called it "Creative Federalism"; maybe the next president will call it "Old Federalism." The point is, this approach is likely to persist in rearing its head regardless of what political party or ideology is presently in vogue, because it makes sense as a counterbalance to ballooning federal control.

One aspect of this approach is an attempt to put more responsibility at the local level to define local needs and priorities. The federal government would set national policies, financing programs in a noncategorical fashion, and probably regulate and evaluate what the local levels are doing with their discretionary funds. The federal government might also provide technical assistance.

Another aspect of this approach is to get out of what was called the "service strategy" of the 1960s and into a "cash strategy." In that period, every time a special interest group identified a new need, such as legal services, food, or whatever, the government would set up a new service program. They would hire professionals to deliver free services, which was 80 percent of the cost right there. About one dollar's worth of service for every fifty dollars spent would get home to the client. Senator Daniel Moynihan of New York in a speech described the service strategy as trying to feed sparrows by first feeding horses.

The cash strategy attempts to give the people the money and let them decide what they want to buy. Rather than set up all these free programs for them to go to, (where they can't get good help anyway) give them the money and let them buy what they want. Many people find it politically unfeasible to give cash to citizens. Others are more paternalistic and feel the poor citizen would make foolish purchases. One variation of the cash strategy is the service voucher. Medicaid is really a voucher. Medical services are bought only by the old and poor who, if they qualify, get to make choices. The general idea would be to assert the philosophy of giving discretionary or semidiscretionary purchasing power to the consumer and let market decisions influence the system. So instead of talking about service *need*, you talk about service *demand*. Instead of a professional coming in and saying: "Three percent of you need speech therapy," you might have a discretionary voucher that allowed you to take it or leave it. Actually only one of you might demand speech therapy. The rest might use the money for family camping because the little speech problem doesn't bother them. Why should we employ speech therapists in free clinics based on what speech therapists say people need?

What's been done so far along these lines? I think general revenue sharing is one approach we know most about in the way of trying to give money to the local county or city with no strings attached except they have to report every quarter how they spend it. It was supposed to give maximum flexibility at the local level. In light of the fact that they also cut back on some of the categorical programs, most mayors feel they have to keep spending the money on some of the same categories that they did before they were cut. Towns have also been reluctant to develop services with general revenue sharing because that usually meant having to hire more civil service personnel, which in turn commits the local government to large fixed expenses overtime. There's no guarantee that general revenue sharing will be continued by Congress. A lot of local governments, therefore, spent their funds at one time on types of purchases, namely equipment or capital construction or improvements. The verdict is still out as to whether or not discretionary dollars at the local level can be translated into flexible and efficient programs for the people in need.

Also, the federal government has tried to strengthen the regional level of federal government through regional councils, whereby regional directors of the various cabinet offices, HEW, HUD, Labor, and so forth, sit together to coordinate programs.

Several times now HEW has introduced the Allied Services Act. Among other provisions this bill would allow the pooling of funds, up to 30 percent of some categorical funds going into a given geographical area, to be redistributed based on local needs and priorities. This bill, however, is not likely to get passed, although I suspect that HEW will continue to seek its passage in future years. It makes too much sense to them for them to just walk away from it.

Another Alternative: Generalists, Unite!

Another approach toward the integration of these fragmented specialized services is through the development of an alliance of generalists. Why would we need such alliance, who would they be, and how would we define such a group?

Consider another analogy: Imagine that these 300 plus categorical programs constitute a plumbing system. Right now there are a lot of encrusted vertical pipelines that go from the top to the bottom. For example, the local school principal is at the bottom of a pipeline of educational program money. He's got a direct line from his school superintendent at the local level who's got a direct line from an assistant superintendent at the state level, who in turn gets his from a commissioner, who knows someone in Washington who knows somebody, and so forth. That's how the money comes down this encrusted pipeline, but there is little or no horizontal plumbing. That local school principal is not interested in the way other funds come into the city, and how or why he might have to share resources with the local director of city parks. It's the same with the professionals in the community mental health centers. They know someone who can get them a grant on their own terms. Why look next door to one's sister agency in rehabilitation to see how you might work together?

There are a lot of vested interest groups from the categorical client through the professionals who are specialists in mental health, education, and welfare. The alliance of generalists would be an alliance of people who could counteract these many groups of powerful specialists.

Specialists are not bad, per se, but they tend to be highly narrow in their view. I'm not saying they aren't vital for service delivery; I *am* saying their power outweighs their contribution! We obviously want and need specially trained personnel at the level of direct service delivery where a transaction of service to a client takes place. But does specialized training in surgery, psychotherapy, or remedial education qualify one to assess the systemic properties of a total delivery system or give one the broader perspective of the multiproblemed family? Who will look out for the interest of the larger system? Who will have sufficient influence or prestige to assess the hidden tradeoffs our society makes whenever we invest millions in a new kidney dialysis machine at the expense of a balanced diet for poor school children? Who cares to think about these choices? Would those who think about them have any strength to shift resources? The generalist is a pretty weak role. Whoever hears a kid say "I want to grow up to be a generalist"? Only through an alliance might a generalist begin to have sufficient influence.

Now who are these generalists who could form an alliance? They might include the elected general officials of town, city, county, and state government, or legislators who, theoretically, do not have a vested interest in a specialized professional type of service. While I also worry about the degree of unselfish integrity in our elected officials, I believe there are many who care. At the very least, these people would have a great legitimacy in claiming to understand what the local needs are, because they are accountable from time to time to a variety of local constituencies and must look for balance among them. At the federal level, the generalists include the regional directors and the regional office staff around the country who do not have categorical program responsibilities.

The alliance could also include various public interest groups such as the U. S. Conference of Mayors, The National League of Cities, the National Association of County Officials, the Council of State Governors, the International City Managers Association, and the various affiliates of these national general purpose organizations. There is also another source, or an associate part of the alliance would be the various United Funds and United Community Service organizations in the private sector that exist in most cities. The generalists include deans in colleges who cannot think about a single discipline. The generalist might include those who are being trained to look at a community and make systemic interventions.

Certainly universities must do more to train generalists. But frankly, most universities are captured and co-opted by the same categorical plumbing system I described before. There are little or no incentives for true interdepartmental collaboration. Beyond the bachelor's degree, it is very difficult to specialize as a generalist.

Let me close this part of my discussion by quoting Seymour Sarason's (1973) book *The Creation of Settings in Future Societies*:

> In the short run, specialization appears to have productive consequences in terms of new knowledge and practice, but in the long run it seems to render the individual, or field, or agency increasingly unable to assimilate and adapt to changes in surrounding social events and processes. Worse yet, the forces (individual and social) which generate specialization unwittingly increase the extent of ignorance of the larger social picture so that assimilation and adaptation are not even perceived as problems.

In other words, it's difficult to tell the categorical specialists that there is a problem because it's likely they're not able to perceive it.

Information Systems as Illustrations of Intergovernmental Affairs

Since the late 1940s, the National Institute of Mental Health (NIMH) has been requiring information on the number of clients seen by mental health treatment facilities. As needs for information have grown, NIMH has aided and encouraged the development of both inpatient and outpatient statistical reporting systems. The traditional audiences for this information have been the state and county governments, which have provided the bulk of the funding for mental hospitals.

With the passage of the Community Mental Health Centers Act in 1963, issues involving continuity of care and responsiveness to community needs have steered the development of information systems in other directions. The needs of administrators and clinicians in decision making about patient care and programs have begun to override considerations of simple statistical reporting. Accountability to both funding sources and recipients of services has placed managers in a position where they can no longer rely on verbal reports of a program's success or annual counts of patients by age and ethnicity. Greater local control and input into the types and quality of mental health services, as well as the more complex daily management tasks posed by comprehensive community mental health centers, require relevant and timely data which must be made available if a program is to survive.

While in theory the task seems simple enough, the dilemmas facing Community Mental Health Centers (CMHC) as they attempt to provide services, as well as evaluate them, are complex. Since CMHC's are mandated to serve a population as part of a comprehensive service network, they must attempt the prevention of mental illness among that population, as well as provide services to those already ill, and must do so as federal funds are gradually withdrawn. Sometimes conflicting demands from state and local officials and citizen boards and the divergent backgrounds of clinical personnel all add to the confusion. A CMHC is frequently caught in the middle and no matter which way it turns, its actions sometimes jeopardize its funding base, its community support, or its base of professional expertise, or possibly all three.

Frequently too, the call for evaluation has provoked the development of elaborate and costly demonstration projects, used on a one-shot basis and geared for esoteric research purposes far removed from everyday patient care or practical management concerns. In the day of secure and generous funding there seemed to be little reason to deviate from this model. Pressures to develop multiple sources of funding as federal programs are scaled down or eliminated have begun to shift the emphasis toward developing sound measures of effort—how much serivce, by what kinds of staff, for how many dollars? This is not to say that issues of efficiency have overwhelmed concerns for effective treatment methods or quality care. Rather the design of systems to measure effort, to measure what is happening now, is the most logical step toward planning for where a program should be in the future, for assessing how quickly programs are meeting their goals, and for evaluating how well these goals meet the needs of the target population.

Management Information System: An Illustration

A management information system (MIS), which can account for the care being given, allows for the determination of costs, track patients to insure continuity of care, provide center managers and staff with data upon which to manage daily operations and to develop long-range goals, cannot but help to increase chances for CMHC survival, growth and effectiveness.

The Greater Lynn Community Mental Health Center is a unit of Union Hospital. For our purpose it is important to note that Union Hospital is also a member of the United Way of Massachusetts Bay (formerly Massachusetts Bay United Fund), the voluntary fund-raising organization for the Metropolitan Boston area.

In the late 1960s and early 1970, my employer, the United Community Planning Corporation of Metropolitan Boston (UCPC is the planning and budgeting arm of the United Fund) gave considerable staff assistance to various agencies in the Lynn area including Union Hospital for the development of both a construction and a staffing grant application to NIMH. Area citizens and other community agency leaders also collaborated in the planning effort that culminated in the application to NIMH. The construction grant was approved and funded. The staffing grant, while approved, was not funded because the federal Office of Management and Budget impounded NIMH funds for those purposes. It was not until 1973 that the funds were released. A major revision of the CMHC staffing grant had to be made, however, due to a cut in funding level, higher personnel costs, and a different philosophy of staffing and program organization that the newly recruited CMHC director brought with him that was not present during the original planning process.

The central office of the CMHC was concerned that whatever system we designed for the Lynn CMHC be capable of providing all information required by the CMHC for fiscal reports, patient status and movement, and staff capabilities and activities. The State of Massachusetts was presently using the Multi-State Information System (MSIS) for its state hospitals. The MSIS did provide some statistical information that the central Department of Mental Health (DMH) offices needed, and while MSIS did not appear to serve the more localized management needs of community-based programs, the central DMH was concerned that any alternative system designed for local management purposes also be able to meet *centralized* DMH needs. The Lynn Area Board was concerned with a wide variety of issues, including specific concerns with what data the system would collect and store, who would control the data, and who would share in the information reports that would be routinely generated. The Lynn Area Board, an official citizens board appointed by the Governor, had been involved in extended negotiations with Union Hospital prior to this time about various aspects of the hospital's fee-for-service contract with the state DMH. While the area board was enthusiastic about the possibilities of an MIS, particularly as it would help them in their functions of program review, evaluation, and planning, they were equally concerned that the costs and efforts to design and operate such a system not detract substantially from the resources available to deliver critically needed services to the general community. After receiving adequate explanations of potentials and limitations, staff of the Lynn Area Board began to formulate the information that they thought the system should generate for the Area Board's purposes.

Another key level of the DMH that had to be involved throughout the project was that of their regional office. Massachusetts is divided into seven major regions and each region is further subdivided into catchment areas. The Lynn CMHC catchment area is located in Region IV. The regional DMH Commissioner was very interested in seeing that an MIS be designed for the Lynn CMHC. He saw an MIS as necessary to evaluate the effectiveness of each DMH-supported program in Region IV but realized that there was not available even the most rudimentary data on services delivered or costs expended.

Most DMH staff and resources for the region were committed to a large state hospital. Some DMH employees who had worked in the former Lynn Area Child Guidance Clinic were delegated by the DMH to work with the union employees of the CMHC staff. These state employees might reasonably be expected in time to also use whatever MIS we designed for use by the Union Hospital staff, although regulations pertaining to state employees did not allow the management of the CMHC to require that they complete the MIS forms unless so ordered by the DMH.

Other government agencies that had to be involved were the national and regional office of NIMH. Whatever system we designed had to be capable of generating the data necessary to answer NIMH reporting requirements. NIMH offices in Washington and the Region I offices in Boston were at the same time very helpful with the provision of documents and technical assistance. The Biometry Branch of NIMH was particularly helpful in providing Series C publications and other reports related to census data use, patient and staff statistics, and management information systems.

You can begin to see here how the information system we were asked to design began to involve us in a number of ways with the various levels of government and the private sector. Besides the various categorical agencies of federal and state governments concerned with mental health, we also had to touch base with the state Executive Offices of Human Services, the state's rate-setting commission, the state's welfare department, and the Attorney General's office. The latter agency had rules and regulations about the confidentiality and patients' rights to access information.

Before describing the overall design of the project, it is important that the reader know of some of the unique features of the Greater Lynn Community Mental Health Center which influenced the direction of the project and the techniques employed by the United Community Planning Corporation staff.

Greater Lynn is made up of five communities about 15 miles north of Boston. Lynn has a significant poverty population and the surrounding four towns are more suburban in nature. The main office and partial hospitalization unit of the CMHC are located at Union Hospital. Construction is presently under way on that site for new inpatient and outpatient facilities.

The overall organizational philosophy of the center is based upon decentralized decision making and leaderless teams. During the first 18 months of its operations, prior to receiving the staffing grant funds, there were only four basic teams: one for prevention education, and two teams providing outpatient care in two separate geographic sections of the catchment area. The two outpatient teams work out of several parttime clinics located in churches and schools throughout the five towns. Each team holds its own weekly meetings and sends a representative to a monthly coordinating meeting. Team members have a great deal of autonomy and work together on a democratic basis without an appointed leader or supervisor other than the center director.

Unlike many other CMHC's, about 40 percent of the center's services are in consultation and education, and there is a large, well-run volunteer program. Volunteers perform a variety of tasks including acting as receptionists at the various clinics, working directly with clients, and participating in indirect services to community groups. Volunteers receive a well-designed orientation and training program. As noted earlier, there are also a number of DMH employees delegated to work under the direction of the CMHC director. These staff work directly in some of the area's schools. While the state employees are under the clinical supervision of the CMHC director, they are administratively responsible to the state DMH and receive salaries based on state pay scales.

With the initiation of the federal staffing grant, the center planned to hire more staff, including a research and evaluation unit and an inpatient service team. When we started our project there were about 30 paid staff, but this number will increase to 100 or more in the near future. Despite its growth, the center director was planning at this point to maintain the decentralized structure and to continue the emphasis on highly mobile teams on community-based clinics. Emergency crisis intervention and indirect services to community agencies would also remain salient.

All of these considerations affected the way we approached the project. We tried to emphasize staff involvement and worked closely with the director and the business manager to insure that our methods were comparable with their philosophy and everyday managements needs.

Project Design

The specific project goal was to assist the Union Hospital-Greater Lynn Community Mental Health Center in designing an integrated management information system which would lend itself to program planning and evaluation, cost-finding and rate-setting, budgeting and daily management. The MIS was to be based upon four subsystems providing data on clients, personnel, programs, and costs. It was to be designed so that it could be transportable to other centers with minimal modification, be compatible with statewide and federal reporting requirements, and yet not infringe upon the client's right to confidentiality.

An informal agreement about the final phases of the project included the development of an environmental monitoring subsystem, a method to routinely collect and analyze information that reflects the social and mental health-related problems and resources of the Lynn catchment area. For example, a method may be designed to routinely compare service statistics of the CMHC with census tract data of the population in the catchment area to point out underserved groups.

The process we used for involving CMHC staff and others in the design and implementation of specific activities was to create three distinct but *integrated* task forces. Each task force was assigned specific subgoals and was assisted by the various UCPC consulting staff.

There were two major requirements in designing a MIS for the Greater Lynn CMHC that led us to adopt a project model utilizing three task forces. As we have previously pointed out, the first and most important of these was the necessity of allowing and encouraging maximum input from the center staff. Experience had shown us that the cooperation and involvement of the people who would be supplying the data for the system was not only desirable but essential if the system were to function. Since the current CMHC staff was small (about 30), it was feasible to include each of them in some direct way in the project.

The second requirement was that some central control over the direction of the project needed to be maintained while subtasks were executed simultaneously. Different members of our staff were therefore delegated responsibility for the work of a single task force, with sufficient leeway to organize the work load and meetings as they saw fit within the project timetable. Coordination was accomplished through a variety of mechanisms, including regular project meetings, informal discussions and the overall supervision of the project by the project manager. In addition, each UCPC project staff member was thoroughly familiar with the goals and activities outlined in the operational plan, thus keeping confusion over roles and tasks to a minimum.

The task forces were considered from the beginning then, as active, working committees and not simply as rubber stamps for a system already completed. Developers of other systems have confirmed our strong belief that staff need to be involved in each phase of MIS design and implementation.

A task force converned with the *client* information subsystem was charged with developing the means to collect the necessary data on clients for the MIS and, at the same time, to satisfy the needs of the clinicians. Members of this task force included the CMHC director and representatives from each team, as well as volunteers and a representative of the Lynn Area Board.

The second task force was primarily concerned with the design of a form to record the services delivered by staff, as well as the time spent on other types of activities.

The fiscal task force, which included the center director, center business manager, hospital comptroller, representatives of the four CMHC treatment teams, the associate area director of the catchment area citizen board, and a staff person from UCPC, was to participate in the design of the fiscal subsystem of the MIS. It was also responsible for recommending the kinds of output reports that should be developed in order that a regular flow of financial data be available for on-going management of the CMHC.

The approach to the task involved two processes: first, meeting with the CMHC business manager and the hospital comptroller to document the existing fiscal procedures the hospital used in operating the CMHC and its capability for handling the enlarged CMHC with its requisite detail; second, working with the task force as a whole to prepare recommendations on the variety of fiscal policy issues with which the CMHC must deal.

The UCPC staff met with representatives of the CMHC and the hospital on three occasions. The first step involved flow chart identification of a typical client entering and passing through the system. This technique was useful in gaining an understanding of the functioning of the CMHC and its relationship to the host organization (hospital). This connection was exemplified by the financial functions carried out by the hospital for the CMHC. Such functions included: (1) the provision of front-end money amounting to $250,000, at one point in time, due to delays in renegotiating the purchase-of-service contract with the state; (2) handling billing functions for all reimbursement situations; (3) providing financial reports to CMHC and hospital management. This review indicated that the hospital was using an accounting system that was adequate for CMHC use and minor changes would allow it to be used for more detailed program accounting by a mental health provider. Also, the hospital was already a participant in a computer-based financial and statistical reporting system with 18 other general hospitals within the state. This participation would not only facilitate operation of the fiscal system but also would offer possibilities for electronic data processing of client and staff activity data. The hospital's highly organized system of financial accountability provided a very substantial base on which to build an integrated management information system.

The next step included the fiscal task force as a whole and began with a meeting that identified the range of issues to be handled. We stressed the importance of the staff's active participation so that the fiscal procedures of the CMHC would be consistent with the program goals of the treatment staff and management. The integrative potentials of a MIS within a CMHC were also reviewed.

At this stage in planning, a tentative decision was made by the hospital and the CMHC that the center would use the hospital's basic accounting system and also that hospital accounting department staff would process all fiscal transactions. At a later time, the CMHC might set up an independent system, which might be more advantageous for purposes of cost finding and rate setting. For the time being, though, the hospital's system would be used.

Reporting forms were required by funding sources. The NIMH Inventory of Community Mental Health Centers is required for annual refunding for staffing grants, and we wanted to be sure the MIS being designed would provide the requisite information. Also, the Commonwealth of Massachusetts Hospital Statement for Reimbursement was reviewed. This is a comprehensive financial statement covering every aspect of hospital activity required by the Massachusetts Rate Setting Commission. This is required since the CMHC is under contract with the state for provision of overhead funds to complement staffing grant funds. It was determined that all required information could be provided by the hospital system when coupled with the MIS under development. The hospital's requirements for contents for CMHC medical records were also established at this time.

The process of designing and implementing an integrated management information system for the Union Hospital-Greater Lynn Community Mental Health Center is not yet completed. The system must be field-tested and the reports produced used by Center staff and management before a success can be claimed. Nevertheless, from our experience with the process today we have every reason to expect success.*

Summary

Without further diversion into the intricacies of the MIS project, let me wrap up by reviewing the major themes I've tried to cover in this chapter.

---

* Author's Note: In mid-1979, the system is fully operational and working well by all reports.

The present service delivery system is highly categorical and consequently inefficient, inaccessible, ineffective for clients with many problems, and generally unmanageable.

There are a number of attempts to integrate these categorical programs at all levels of government, ranging from national legislation, changes in federal bureaucracy or regulations, through changes in state and local government structure. Many attempts are being made to integrate services at the level of the direct service agencies.

Intergovernmental relationships are becoming increasingly complex, and they are not likely to be simplified in the near future. Human service planners must work as generalists to cut across levels of government and the vertically designed categorical program structure. To be effective, generalists at all levels must begin to forge alliances with one another.

Some extremely important technological innovations, such as information systems can be used to help integrate services, as well as make them more accountable and subject to subsequent effectiveness evaluation. The design and implementation of such systems, however, will require the skills of generalists if the systems are not to simply reinforce the existing weaknesses of the categorical service delivery.

THE CONTINUING EFFORT TO CHALLENGE OLD WAYS AND TO ASSESS PROGRESS

The chapters of the preceding section reveal many of the problems and frustrations of administering human services in a context of political and economic forces, and show how some good things can happen in spite of our efforts to make them happen. They also show how hard it is to bring about improvements in the way things are.

We will see more of that in this section but in the context of evidence that ingenuity as well as hope "springs eternal" in the breasts of people dedicated to making things better for people who are retarded, mentally ill, old and decrepit, young and rebellious, or just not able to make it in modern society. We may also hope or despair (depending on one's point of view) that we are making progress in our ability to find out what the effects of human services actually are.

Yes, our institutional ways of delivering human services do appear to be relatively rigid, as seen by their critics, and defensive of how they do what they were set up to do. But they do not, contrary to their critics, resist all efforts at improvement. Changes do take place, though sometimes slowly, and not as a result of overpowering political pressure or administrative edict. The public schools do innovate, and do this with the cooperation of outsiders, if those outsiders are competent enough to understand the school and the needs of its staff. Some evidence of this is.shown in the lessons reported by a community psychologist seeking to help a school develop a better general climate for learning. And those lessons can be generalized, again, if the practitioner wants to learn from them.

People in some institutions where they are treated as sick and made dependent on professionals who would administer healing treatments need not always have institutionalized "treatment" in their futures. Different ways of perceiving mentally retarded children and emotionally disturbed people are emerging. By seeking changes in individual behavior (and that too is not easy) through means called educational rather than medical treatment, we are able to open a new set of opportunities for human care and create new attitudes toward people with problems. A child with learning difficulties need not be labeled as a retardate and thus placed indefinitely in a dependent relation with others, usually strangers in some special school or hospital; he might just as well be left to the care of his family when they have been taught how to care for him and possibly educate him toward less dependence. They themselves could then take pride in a successful assumption of responsibility.

Likewise, the mentally or emotionally disturbed need not be seen exclusively as sick and in need of medical attention. After all, most behaviors that are problems to someone were learned somewhere along the course of a person's growth and development. Why can't they be unlearned and others substituted for them? An educational model of behavior change toward self-reliance can reasonably supplant a medical model which too often puts the individual in a dependent relation to an "expert"—a relationship that usually does the individual little good and is often very hard to break. Rationales and some supporting research for these different ways of conceiving problem behaviors are summarized.

Finally, we return to the persistent question: Is all of this— whether old or new—doing any good? Today's legislative and bureaucratic emphasis on accountability has created a demand for more rational, reliable, and immediate answers. As one result, a whole new field of applied social technology, evaluation, has emerged. It is based on recent developments in social measurement, the growing sophistication in systems analysis and in defining goals, benefits, and costs. Program evaluation is welcomed by many, such as administrators and legislators feeling a need for less ambiguous means of telling their constitutents how much good they are doing (or how badly the competing program is faring), and by social scientists of many ilks who would enjoy the benefits of a new industry. Others are less enthusiastic, fearing that a new numerology can be used as a more refined way to hoodwink the public with statistics, and generally worried that too detailed knowledge of social process can become an oppressive tool some day in the wrong hands. The community is just better for having services, some argue, never mind whether they are really efficient or businesslike. Some of these issues and new technologies in the evaluation process are explored in later parts of this section.

Uncommon common sense is one way of summarizing the important ingredients of successful mental health consultation in communities. James Kelly reports his personal experience over six years of doing community mental health work through the schools of a Michigan city. Among the commonsensical ideas coming from this experience is a positive view of people as resources upon which to build relationships rather than casualties to be repaired. Starting from here and then demonstrating that each community has its own unique qualities, Kelly shows why efforts to bring about change must attend to the multiple social and political forces of the community. That it takes more than one kind of skill, and ideas from many professions and disciplines to devise a workable intervention is illustrated as Kelly describes the difficulty of translating this evident platitude into lasting and self-sustaining action programs.

Chapter 15

SOME "LEARNINGS" FROM DOING COMMUNITY WORK

James G. Kelly

I am going to present five ideas derived from my personal experiences in doing community work. These ideas are offered as premises for thinking about the qualities of persons and social situations. I hope that the ideas are useful in improving the effectiveness of community groups and for improving the personal and professional development of those doing community work.

Persons as Resources

This idea is a very difficult one to implement, particularly for psychologists. The conceptual framework, the work settings, and the concepts of psychology have historically emphasized deficiencies and sickness. While this frame of reference is appropriate for the treatment of persons who are not functioning adequately, it is grossly inadequate when working at the community level; most of the persons with whom community work will be done have talents and skills that are essential for seeing a community program through to completion. The challenge is to find and involve skillful and talented persons. If the view of persons emphasizes limitations, deficiencies, and foibles, we can easily overlook talent that is not visible and striking. I believe very strongly that a working premise for carrying out community work should include a conception of persons in the worker's mind that embraces personal and technical competencies.

I can remember very well learning this point firsthand. In 1960, my colleagues and I began to develop an intervention program in an elementary school that focused on providing multiple services for nonachieving children. The particular program included an evaluation design for a special class for nonachieving children. The services were a group discussion program on child rearing for parents of the children, a home visitation program for the mothers, and a consultation program to the classroom teacher. The principal of the school in this particular case had had very little involvement in the creation and design of the program. He had inherited this innovative idea spawned by outside professionals and the central school administration. When I began to visit the school as the consultant, he was never in his office, he was busy elsewhere in the building and created many different ways to avoid contact with me. I began to make sure that the school secretary had a working knowledge of what a consultant did and relied on her for the first two weeks to understand the purpose of the program and to communicate her impressions to the principal.

One day when my coat was in a locker and the secretary had gone home, I was forced to seek out the principal in a distant part of the building. I asked him for his help in retrieving my coat. On that long walk back to the principal's office, he and I began to establish rapport and gradually over time the school principal began to see the program (and me) as a useful resource. During those first two weeks, however, there were a lot of ideas in my head, a lot of hypotheses about why the principal was avoiding and resisting me and the program. I began to think about the principal in ways which put him down, minimizing his contribution. I began to think of him as recalcitrant, obstinate, evasive, anxious, and a personally threatened person. I even imagined him as not very competent as a school principal. I know somehow that such ideas were not fair and perhaps wrong. I persisted in making contact, to give him feedback over the phone, until the night I had to ask for his help in retrieving my coat.

A year later, I talked with him about my early entry into his school, and I shared with him my concerns and frustrations as I could recall them. I asked him if he could recall how he felt and thought during that time. His response was that two years before my coming to the school a psychologist had come to him and told him that he could help him. What the psychologist was going to do was to improve the climate of the first-grade classroom. What happened was that the psychologist turned the classroom into a group therapy program, with the result that the educational program quickly went out the window. The children in the classroom were boisterous, noisy, and completely out of control. They were destructive of physical property in and outside of the room, and they spent much of their time in the hallways distracting other children. The psychologist was definitely not helping; worse, he was designing a large nuisance.

The school principal said that when he saw me I represented another psychological nightmare. The best thing he could do, he said, was to wait to see what I would do. He was not enthusiastic to help until I proved by myself that I did something other than what his experience had been of what a psychologist does. He also indicated that he felt psychologists read minds, and he did not want his mind to be read by me.

I can vividly recall this experience today! What it meant to me is that whenever a community worker enters a new setting, the people in that setting respond to the stronger both with the experiences they had with similar persons, as well as their fantasies about who that person is. However unfounded, however untested, however personal such experiences and fantasies are, they provide the context for the worker. It may be that caution or skepticism that is often present in response to an outsider is an adaptive community response. What is important is that the community worker should not respond with a point of view or a set of concepts that describes such tentativeness as pathologic. What the community worker must do is to keep testing out how a new relationship can be built so that the talents, the skills, and the competencies of the people can be determined, and how the resources of the community worker can be contributed to the community. A potential asset of psychological training for community work is the care and attention to the sensitivity of interpersonal relationships; one of the handicaps of psychological training for community work is the tendency to categorize difficulty as pathologic. A personal hallmark for me is to learn how to think about persons as resources rather than as casualties.

Communities Do Vary from Place to Place

This sounds like a truism that we don't pay much attention to. In order to cope with the vast variety and confusion in designing an innovative program, there is an imperative need to develop some ideas that will help us illuminate the confusion and say, "Ah, yes, that's the same kind of confusion I saw before." There's a tendency to look at every community social system with an effort to extract generalities. I argue, however, that no matter how much experience we have in any one community or how many different communities we work in, we can expect unique variations that will produce new topics for debate and new political constraints affecting any imposed intervention. There will be new rites of passage for the person trying to develop a program. This is a humbling reality. I assert that no matter how good and how effective we were in the last community, there's likely to be new and different demands on us in our current community. If we succeed in our current community work, we will learn still newer and different ideas and ways of adapting that may or may not be useful for the next occasion.

The implication of this idea is not to strive to be clever, or a person for all settings, but to realize that every community demands a different type of organizational structure for innovative programs and personal and political resources to cope effectively with uniqueness. What is also useful is a point of view that encourages different ways to look at community topics and events that illustrate the unique.

In order to design an effective preventive program for different communities, the community worker will adapt to the community variations and conditions. This process of personal adaptation by the community worker produces much stress and requires an aggressive and persistent effort to understand how our own views of the community, our own personal values, and our own interpersonal skills can be enlarged and expanded in order to cope with the unique demands placed upon us when doing community work at this time and in this place.

I can again recall clearly the awareness of this principle of community variation when working with six elementary schools in a very rural, satellite community in the Detroit metropolitan area. Each of the elementary schools was serving persons with roughly similar social and class backgrounds. The social dynamics of each one of the elementary schools was unique, and each school within the same community was unique to itself. Over time, each mental health consultant to the six schools was required to adapt to the unique culture of each school. The mental health program was developed for each school while offering mental health consultation to the faculty and principal, to provide better diagnostic and mental health services for the children. Each program operated with its own pace, style, and direction, created out of the historical relationships between principal and teacher, and out of the parental values, parental concern, and competences and interests of the consultant. It was also expected that the program would help stimulate a more organized effort by the entire school system to improve mental health services for children in that community.

Over a six-year period, from 1966 to 1972, two of the six elementary schools developed what could be interpreted as a quality and effective mental health program. In one school, the parents, the principal, and the faculty developed a multiservices center within the school building, where mothers came to classes on child rearing, and where the school became a community center for recreation and social services, including a day care center. The second successful school focused on the education and training of parents as teacher aides and thus as educational resources for the school building. The other four elementary schools never really developed a community-based, parent-involved mental health program for children or faculty. While all four schools did have the services of school building consultants over the six-year period, they never did get off the ground. A one-third success rate seems admirable, in retrospect, given the host of personal, social, organizational, economic and political events that impede attaining program implementation.

In thinking about the ingredients contributing to the programs in these two schools, I come up with the following. In the two successful schools, the principals had a clear, unyielding commitment to serve the community. This commitment could be relied and depended upon by faculty, parents, and consultants to support development of services to the community. These two school principals were not necessarily the best educators, but they were certainly the most committed elementary principals. Second, in both schools, there was a visible and consistent rapport between the tenured and nontenured teachers. Somehow the status differentials latent in the hierarchical social system were not barriers for the development of a school program. There was indeed adequate informal communication and respect by both tenured and nontenured teachers for each other. Third, there was in the community a handful of committed, interpersonally competent parents who were persistent in their efforts to improve the quality of education in "their" school. Fourth, the consultants who worked in these two schools were persons who understood and applauded the teachers, the principal, and the parents as people. They were able to go beyond their own professional roles as experts and develop rapport and a genuine relationship that added an extra dimension to the quality of the school environment.

The lessons I learned from this six-year expedition in designing a school mental health consultation program are: (1) there are definite contextual constraints in affecting the success of community-based programs; (2) what is important is to examine in each locale how the combination of resources—personal, political, and economic—can be brought together to develop a community program that has both useful and lasting impact. After six years of work, two schools did it. Those were the schools that had commitment for community programming expressed by the school administration, the teaching faculty, the parents, and the consultant. These schools provided an opportunity to go beyond the formal roles of teacher, administrator, parent and consultant which resulted in a congealing effort with an outside consultant to persevere and deliver a quality program.

Multiple Social and Political Strata of the Community

There are traditions for each profession that focus upon ways of thinking and work methods that define how a member of a profession solves a problem. These ways of thinking and preferred methods of work for each profession also create limitations when any one discipline or profession solves a community problem or develops a community program. Community work does not coincide with a disciplinary perspective. It is my experience that most tough problems such as problems of inadequate service delivery and racial and sex discrimination, are problems that cannot be solved by any one profession or any one set of techniques or concepts.

The validity of multiple points of view is twofold. One is that each profession brings unique ideas and approaches to the solution of problems. The second is that each discipline increases the possibility of impacting on those parts of the community's social structure that must be involved if a solution is created, developed and tried out. The psychological bias of only looking at the individual or only looking at psychological variables produces short-lived interventions. In my experience, many of the factors that contribute to disorganization at the personal or social level in a community are forces that are not psychological in nature. The community traditions, the cultural values of people and their communities, plus the distribution of wealth, job discrimination of the political structure, etc., reduce the possibility that persons of low social status or low economic livelihood will have impact in decision making. Social and community interventions should be designed so as to include multiple political and social strata of the community.

In the community described above, where there was an active effort to develop a school mental health program in six elementary schools, the school principal and the classroom teachers were the consultees. Whenever there was a question raised inside or outside the school systm about the real utility of the service, the answer was effective to the extent that our staff understood the social organization of the school system. We made very active efforts to maintain continuous communication with the teachers' union, with the superintendent, with the school board, with parent advisory groups, with the janitorial staffs, and with the community leaders who did not have children in the school system. We consciously related to persons at different social strata, beyond our immediate consultees. The willingness of key, influential citizens and school administrators to financially support the school mental health program was related to the efforts we made in problem solving and assisting such relevant resources. We expanded our efforts to define our usefulness. In my opinion, the maintenance of the mental health program and related community development activities in that community could not have been maintained without a sensitivity to the ongoing relationships with key, multiple social strata in the particular community. We took to heart the axiom that knowing the territory is essential and that organized staff resources must be able to respond to unplanned crises.

One important event came about as a result of the consultative relationship to the school superintendent. He was concerned about the competences of his administrative staff. One of the consultation sessions focused upon a particular person he was considering promoting to a higher level administrative post. I expressed to him that while I had no firm basis to offer an opinion, I had an uneasy feeling that the person he had in mind for the promotion did not have the psychological maturity and make-up to withstand much stress. There was something about his interpersonal relationships that I didn't quite understand. I hoped that he would pay particular care when evaluating the person. This person was the focus of conversations between the superintendent and myself over several months. Very late in the evening, the superintendent called me at home and said that he would take my advice from now on. The shocking validity of my concern was that the person had molested a child who was an elementary student in the school system. The repercussions and political consequences of having a member of the educational profession behave in such a way was potentially catastrophic and shocking to the system. The superintendent and I began at once an active effort to get help for the person, to initiate planning to replace this particular individual, and to help coach the administrative staff, teaching faculty, and school board to take immediate and positive actions.

As I look back, my vague, diagnostic concerns and the unfortunate validity they were given was a primary factor in support of the mental health program in the school system. The superintendent saw a very real example of the potential usefulness of a school consultation program as a result of the conversations I had with him and my efforts to focus upon a careful assessment of teaching staff. While the efforts did not prevent an unfortunate occurrence, the superintendent respected the validity and earnestness of mental health consultation.

While this example is extreme, my guess is that any type of community or social intervention program will succeed as a result of similar unplanned demonstrations of help. It's not enough to be professionally competent and to deliver a quality program. The program staff must establish support for community programs at multiple levels of that system. Over the six-year period we had similar examples of our staff assisting the teachers' union, parent advisory groups, the school board, and county commissioners. When push came to shove, a cross-section of clients, school administrative staff, elective officials, and influential citizens knew enough about who we were and what we did and could do, that they could support the program. It is clear to me now that no long-term community program can flourish without active, persistent work with the multiple strata of the community. Doing this means that we have a chance to be in the right place at the right time.

Many Ideas and Skills Are Needed for the Creation of a Workable Intervention

The tough social issues demand that knowledge, expertise, opinions, and good will go beyond any one discipline. It is likely that work will be more effective if the program staff works at multiple levels of the community and if it includes persons of different disiplinary heritages and points of view.

There is another, perhaps even more important, reason for having community work sponsored by persons with-multiple disciplines. Persons available wth different professional and technical competences minimize the risk of working in the community through the biases and the myopia of any one discipline. Psychologists are particularly vulnerable to believing that psychological knowledge can make a difference in the quality of community life or that psychological knowledge per se can reduce the prevalence of social and community problems. There are numerous examples in the literature of social and community interventions where the combination of psychological and economic interventions can produce some substantial, long-term results (Kelly, Snowden & Munoz, 1976). There are examples where the relationship between psychological expertise in recreation and leisure activities can make a difference for the improvement of community life and well-being. It is my belief that students in psychology interested in community work need the opportunity to work on community problems in conjunction with students in other disiplines (Kelly, DiMento & Gottlieb, 1972). I would like to believe also that students in other disciplines find something useful in a psychological perspective.

In the community I've mentioned above, it became clear in carrying out our consultation program that the consultation to junior high school classroom teachers would not impact unless recreational opportunities for the junior high school age population could be provided in that community. Through the combined work of graduate students at the University of Michigan in architecture and urban planning, proposals were developed for using open space for recreational purposes and for creating a relatively low-cost, recreational park located on the physical property of the junior high school. The process of planning that activity in conjunction with the parents, high school faculty, and the county and township recreation departments highlighted the notion that adequate recreational space can be related to the promotion of mental health, particularly in a community that is geographically isolated, had a very low tax base, and that has no previous commitment to use land for youth recreation. As the recreational program design was identified with the mental health consultation program, students and faculty in the junior high school again became aware that mental health consultants could be useful, could get down to work on a real problem, and have some direct payoffs in promoting a good climate in the junior high school.

When we started the school mental health consultation program, there was no expectation that we would become involved in the design of recreational programs. It became apparent however, that without attention to the recreation and leisure needs of the junior high school age student, we would be operating a mental health program that was short-sighted, incomplete, and invalid. One of the side benefits of this phase of the program was that the graduate students in community psychology who were involved in learning about mental health consultation became strong advocates for a multi-disiplinary approach to community work. With this new axiom, it was believed by all of us that we were really becoming serious and useful about solving a community problem and not just selecting community work to correspond with our vested interests. We began to feel that multi-disciplinary collaboration may have a long-term impact for the well-being of the community.

Community Work Involves a Commitment to Personal Growth and the Creation of a Supportive Culture

Community problems lie beyond the usual boundaries of disciplinary competence. The solution of community problems also involves going beyond our traditional training. Working to solve community problems means we have to put our real selves into the solution which make us vulnerable for failure. In this work, we increase the probability that our investment in disciplinary training may be invalid, or limited, because what we know how to do doesn't work. Working on community problems generates a Gargantuan amount of ambiguity. We can never be sure at any one time where our political support is, where the real problem lies, and often how best to go about solving it. The tensions created by being vulnerable to risk, by continuing to question our basic professional and personal identity, requires a new kind of working relationship among colleagues doing community work. In fact, good community work requires an active, ongoing cultural support system. This, itself, is a difficult assignment because most professional training programs do not encourage the creation of such support systems. The presence of such support systems is not believed to be critical as a criterion for training programs.

    In the process of working with a multidisciplinary team of professionals in psychiatry, social work and psychology, as well as with students who were becoming professional in those fields, I have become convinced that this is an essential criteria for training. In the training program I have referred to above, it was initially very hard to have social workers support psychologists and psychologists support psychiatrists in doing mental health consultation. It was very difficult for the established professional to admit failure and to applaud the good work of a student. It was difficult to develop a social setting where communication could be direct, constructive, with the goal of improving the competence of the person involved.

It is my own belief, however, that the success of the school consultation program, both as a training program and an educational program, was related to those occasions where the qualities of persons involved were allowed free reign in spite of social status, disiplinary training, political values, and previous community experience.

There *were* occasions when a multidisciplinary group of people who previously had been strangers could function as a resource network. Those occasions were not as often as I would have liked, but they did occur frequently enough to serve as an invisible, congealing force allowing us to think out loud when we had bumbled, and to applaud each other when we perceived success.

These five observations are offered as ideas I believe important for insuring quality community work. I didn't start out my work with these ideas in mind. The lessons I have learned were learned as a result of an active effort to try to develop social and community interventions that are preventive, are supported by citizens, and that have sustained impact. When I think about these lessons, they sometimes appear as common sense. If they are, what professional training needs is more of the "uncommon" common sense.

The point has been made that to deinstitutionalize means the capacity to normalize the individuals from either the point of view of preventing institutionalization or of bringing someone back into the community or family. The need to normalize and means of normalizing those labeled mentally retarded is discussed in detail from the point of view of a man involved with the successful development and implementation of a self-help program for the parents of retarded persons. Beneath the cool and lucid exposition of the program, there is a depth of personal commitment that could only explain the care and perseverance required to carry the project through. Here is a beneficient use of behavior modification that steers clear of the brave new world.

Chapter 16

ALTERNATIVES TO INSTITUTIONALIZING A MENTALLY RETARDED CHILD: A SELF-HELP PROGRAM FOR PARENTS AND CHILD

Bruce L. Baker

The Retarded and the Institutions: Some Figures

About 80 percent of the people who are called retarded also have another label, cultural familiar retardation, which in effect means that their retardation is the result of the kind of living conditions under which they grew up. This is where poverty, racism and poor schools contribute in a large part to their retardation. Only about 20 percent of the retarded are genuinely organically retarded for some reason or other; 95 percent of the people called retarded live at home; only 5 percent live in institutions. I think that is an interesting fact, because institutionalism and deinstitutionalization is very much in the news and we hear a lot about it. It's very big in Pennsylvania, because this is where a lot of the important early class action suits took place.

One of the reasons why there is such concern for deinstitutionalization is that 95 percent of the money in the field of retardation goes to the 5 percent of the people in the institutions because these large-scale institutions are enormously expensive to maintain. *Mainly* because of the cost problems, there's an increasing sophistication now towards getting people out of institutions, and the movement in this country is modeled in philosophy, although not necessarily in practice, after the move in the Scandinavian countries.

Normalization

I don't know how many of you are familiar with the normalization principle and the kinds of deinstitutionalization movement that's taken place in Scandinavia, but it is a fascinating movement. It cannot be translated into the United States, in part, because of the political differences of the two settings. In Scandinavia, people are generally cared for by the state from birth until death so that a very comprehensive system in the field of retardation is just similar to the comprehensive system one finds in every other field. The overriding philosophy in living for the retarded is a philosophy known as *normalization.*

The philosophy is essentially that one should create for the retarded as normalized an environment as possible, so that a retarded individual can lead as normal a life as possible, but also an environment that in some ways respects the retarded's right to be different. So that, in Scandinavia, there's been a great concentration on architectural design of physical living facilities that are not just like the facilities other people live in but are aimed at making the retarded people as normal as possible. They may not always look exactly the same as other people, but they look as much the same as possible, given the people's handicaps, and they try to gear all their intentional training from age one to making a person more and more able to live some sort of a normal life.

The reason that this does not translate readily in the United States is that we don't have all of the various support services. Thus, when one talks now about deinstitutionalizing the retarded in this country, and setting up a bunch of very normalized kinds of community living facilities, many of the retarded are not at all prepared to take advantage of those because they haven't had the prior training.

Nevertheless, the community residence movement has really taken off. It has become a very big movement in Massachusetts where the Governor is committed to deinstitutionalizing 3000 persons over the next four years. Simultaneously, Massachusetts has become committed to the small group home model, which is defined as having a maximum of nine retarded people and three staff living together in a small facility. Now if you divide 9 retarded people into the 3000 deinstitutionalized, one begins to envision a network of about 400 of these small group homes cropping up across Massachusetts, all of which, according to the Massachusetts state plan, will look the same.

It doesn't take a great deal of sophistication to know that that's absurd, and about a year ago, some of my students and I said, "Look, there are lots of different options that Massachusetts could be considering and is not. Why don't we propose to do a basic demographic survey of all the various kinds of community living arrangements that are available for the retarded across the country and then see if we can develop for Massachusetts a little more systematic state plan as to how it might broaden its vision a bit?" So through the Massachusetts Developmental Disabilities Council, we are now running the only evaluation program of the state, and we're doing that in two stages. We're looking through questionnaires about community residences all across the country and through some intensive eight-day, live-in visits at fifteen different models in the Northeast.

The model I'm most excited about is in Pennsylvania, specifically, the transitional services model in Pittsburgh. It is a huge, privately run model housing 500 retarded people. Anyway, we have identified 15 different models, all of which the state of Massachusetts should in some way be considering as options.

Incidentally, we found over a thousand different community residences across the country for the retarded. This is becoming a big movement that has no intercommunication at the moment. But one of the indices that we were interested in was the flow through these settings. The turnover rate is such that a bed is filled every two years, so that people do not go in, at least at the moment, until these facilities are stagnant. That's in part because the earliest people to move out of institutions are those who could most capably function in the community anyway.

So we will probably begin to see some differences in the next couple of years in terms of the turnover rate. Almost a quarter of the people go into the facilities and then fall back into the institutions. Traditionally, research in this field has tried to look at those individual characteristics of people that predict whether they will make it in the community, however, the reason that most of these people do or don't make it has to do with the kinds of facilities that are available in their setting. Often, the very same person who could make it in a small group home would fail miserably in a semi-independent apartment arrangement and vice versa. Someone who would do well in a semi-independent apartment is too high functioning for a small group home with house parents, doesn't like it, won't stick with the mundane, sheltered, workshop kind of job, becomes a big problem to everybody, and ends up back in the institution.

Different parts of the country have different models. For instance, Rhode Island has just a semi-independent apartment model. So if someone comes out of the state institution in Rhode Island, and they can't function without a full-time staff on the round, they go back to the institution. Massachusetts has just a small group home model; Vermont is using foster care. A pretty comprehensive service is needed for the retarded, not only for the adults but also for children both to develop the whole bag of requisite skills that one needs to function in the community, and to provide a whole different array of possible living arrangements in the community.

This leads me indirectly to what we're doing, because if you talk to people about the community residence movement, they all say, "My God, why should an institution need to be toilet training or teaching time skills or money skills or transportation skills? Why didn't the parents teach them this stuff?" And, in fact, now that there is such a press against putting people into institutions, and they're staying at home, parents have become very vocal in saying, "Well, if I'm going to keep my retarded child at home, what will I do?" My colleagues and I have become very interested in the last several years in education or training for parents to become a part of that service delivery system. There are a lot more parents than professionals, therefore, it makes sense to train the parents in the care of their retarded child.

Parent Education and Behavior Modification

One of the political implications that we were concerned with when we started doing parent education was that it could be misinterpreted as implying that the responsibility lies with the parents and that the state doesn't have a responsibility to provide services. Consequently, we've been very concerned all along with not only looking to see where the parents can develop skills and help their kids at home, but what that does to the parents as advocates for services in the community. What happens in fact is that the more effective you make parents, the more effective advocates they also become in pressing for services.

The research I'm going to discuss here is a convergence of several trends. One is the trend toward parent education and the other is toward the use of more behaviorally oriented methods in the home mental health field or in dealing with the retarded. Behavior modification is simply an intervention approach which looks at observable direct behaviors. This is a better intervention approach to consider in dealing with the retarded than intervention approaches that look at interpsychic social conflicts and structures and deal at an ethereal level because many of the retarded kids do not function at an ethereal level all that much, but they do have descriptive behavior that can be observed and analyzed. So that the behavior modification approach has tried to take a lot of basic learnings of experimental psychology, not necessarily learning theory, and translate those into things that one might do to help (in this case) a retarded child learn more. It's definitely an educational treatment approach as opposed to a medical treatment approach. And it's very much concerned with the relationship between a person and the setting that he or she is in.

What it does, then, is to translate into a whole series of techniques that modify different environments so that the press of the environment is more towards adaptive behavior and that the consequence of that behavior is something that essentially strengthens it and makes it more likely to reoccur. In programming for the retarded, people have begun to take a look at the whole person in relationship to the state institutional ward that he's living in or the home environment. They are looking at some of the things about this environment that effectively make someone function in a more retarded way and some of the ways that we can both change some of the antecedents and also the results of the behavior so that not only is a more normalized behavior more likely to occur, but the behavior is strengthened as a result of its consequences. Although a whole series of techniques evolve from that, often you'll hear them identified with behavior modification. Some techniques are good, some are bad, some are useful for one person and totally irrelevant for another, some are more ethical than others, and so on.

In this particular series, we took a relatively new approach which appears to be fairly simpleminded and at least is very easy to train nonprofessionals in and introduce it to parents. It's a very recent movement; the parent-training behavior model only goes back about 10 years, and really not more than 5. Most of the early studies were single case where a highly motivated, quite middle-class family would bring their retarded child into the psychologist's office and work with him intensively by observing the child being taught through one-way mirrors, videotape feedback, and communication by "bug-in-the-ear" devices. This is very costly but effective in getting parents to then carry some techniques over into the home and teach survival skills to their children.

Over the last couple of years the question of reducing the cost and extending the service to more families has been raised. One way is to use nonprofessional trainees, or, what we set out to do, was develop training packages so that a parent does not need a professional there at all.

Designing a Training Package for Parents

We did a survey of families with retarded children aged about 3 to 15 and asked them what some of their priorities were. What were some things that really bugged them around the house that they would like to see changed? Predictably, the first most important item is toilet training, followed by tense behavior problems, other self-help skills, speech and communications skills, and finally what we call play skills to keep the child active.

What we decided to do is to take our knowledge of behavior modification and package it into a series of manuals that could teach parents how to deal with their child in any of those different skill areas, and also that would be written at various child levels. So that, ideally, one could give any parent an appropriate manual, depending on the child's level, that would help the parent develop his or her own programs. It also has colored pages which give very brief one- or two-page outlines on how to teach such things as spreading butter with a knife, eating with a fork, taking a bath, setting a table, the kinds of community-living skills that a child needs to learn.

We developed 10 manuals. Some help speech, play, and behavior control; in some of these areas, we developed a whole series. They have fun illustrations, and the programs are very short. Similar packages have been developed by teaching programs which take a very different approach. They try to develop such a highly structured program that nothing is left to chance. Ours is very different. No parents have used our programs in exactly the way they have been written, because the manual points out repeatedly that the parent has already taught the child a great deal and that these are just general guidelines.

Testing the Training Package Design

One of the first things we did was test the general packaging approach. Early in the program we sent a group of 47 parents an assesment manual saying, in effect, "If you're interested in taking part in this thing, send us back the assessment." And then we started to do a branching study of how many people responded and how many did not: 25 people responded; 22 didn't. Of those who did, we did some follow-up and got an additional 11 respondents. Then, within the manual we had a system where you send back a postcard when you started teaching, and we got very few respondents on that. It was a very small number, only about 5 of the 47 people did the whole process all by themselves without any coercion.

After spending about a year developing these manuals, we studied them in the largest parent-training study that's been done in behavior modification. We used 160 families. The family had to live within a 20-mile radius of Boston and have a retarded child who was functioning somewhere within the range of our manuals. We met the families in several large group sessions, gave them an introduction to the study, and told them exactly what the various experimental conditions were: 20 percent would be assigned randomly to a control condition to do pretest measures at a 4-month interval followed by treatment or training. These people knew that they were going to be controls. Another 20 percent of the parents were assigned to each of four experimental conditions.

The first group was given the manuals, turned on their own for 4 months, kept daily logs which they mailed to us, but received no feedback on the logs. This was terrible behavior modification strategy, but was obviously the cheapest condition. The next group had the manuals *plus* biweekly phone calls that were structured, lasted about a half an hour, and taught the parents about how their teaching was going in specific terms. This is very typical of the model that's used now, especially in rural areas where people live a long distance from the clinic. It is used a lot by visiting nurses and social workers now to maintain phone contact with parents. The third technique was to have parents use the manuals again, but also have biweekly group sessions in groups of eight families with two group leaders. A series of nine group meetings was held for training in behavior modification. This is a typical training device that's being used across the country.

The final one was groups plus home visits. This has only been used experimentally since it costs so much. These folks have the manuals and a group meeting every 2 weeks, and on alternate weeks they have a psychologist or one of our staff go into their home, model for them, watch what they were doing with their child, and give them on-the-spot consultation.

What we have here is a series of perceptual involvements, and the kinds of questions we are asking are as follows: First of all, can parents learn and do behavior modification when they have nothing but written and instructional materials? What are the immediate effects of the programs they carry out and what are some of the generalized effects on their child? What are the results of increased professional support? How much benefit is there from more expensive conditions? What are the participation rates in this kind of business? What are the drop-out rates? What correlates with or predicts drop out and what generally predicts success?

This is the first study large enough to do multiple regression analysis on dependent variables and take a look at what parent characteristics or child characteristics might predict success under various conditions. In the mental health field there has been very little of that done. Very rarely are data gathered to assist in placement, treatment, and so on. More often the patient has to match the clinic's orientation, whether it is client-centered psychoanalytic, and so on.

Of the families that began training, 87 percent completed. Of those, 78 percent completed the postmeasures. We lost a few families in the process of postmeasures. The average attendance at group sessions on these two conditions was 90 percent. We didn't have a lot of problems motivating parents.

The measure that we developed over the last 4 years of how much parents learn about behavior modification principles correlates somewhat with actual practice. But a big problem that we're working on is to try to get a measure of practice and knowledge that correlate in some way. It's at least a necessary, if not sufficient, condition to being able to do something with your child. You have to know some of the basic teaching principles. Our measure plots change points to control groups of the various treatment conditions. In this training experience, the highest change overall came in the mothers in the manual-only condition. In an overall analysis, every one of these changes was significantly different from zero; and every one of these treatment conditions was significantly different from the controls for the mothers. But the most significant for the mothers was in the manuals-only, the least in the phone call. This finding will replicate time after time. The best results in terms of what they actually learn about the process came to most people who had no professional help at all. They were completely on their own. The worst was in those people who had special help, but no face-to-face contact.

I should point out a couple of things about the controls: 95 percent of all these children went to school. So, when we look at child measures and find significant differences in the controls, we have to remember that they were in school for that 4-month period. The differential effect is perhaps 15 minutes of extra work a day with the child beyond the huge amount of schooling that they get. We discovered something with the control parents. In our kick-off meeting, we gave parents a basic general introduction to behavior modification. They still got a pre- and postassessment of their child. The assessment is 28 pages of specific behavioral assessment that many parents found incredibly valuable. It was really the most intensive behavioral assessment they'd ever had of their child, and what we had later was a lot of controls who reported, "that assessment was terrific. I never thought I'd teach him to cut meat with a knife. As soon as I read that, I went out and taught him that." And in fact a lot of teaching took place not because of the specific principles, but because parents just started exposing their kids to other stimuli. One-third of our control group joined another behavior modification group, where they read books and articles, and they did something as a result. But they shouldn't have been doing it if they had been good experimental subjects; but this was the real world, and if they heard that there was a technique that might help their child, they just went out and learned the technique anyway.

Most of our planning is geared towards self-help skills, by which we mean a whole range of skills in grooming, dressing, eating, and housekeeping—a whole range of patterns of daily living skills that one might teach a child when he or she is 15. Every parent took off to teach on the average of about four or five different skills during the course of 4 months.

Our behavioral problem manual is not as specific as the self-help manual. Behavioral problems usually relate in terms of the way parents and their children interact. Sometimes another objective observer coming in and taking a look at that can be extraordinarily helpful. I was talking to a behavior modifier on the West Coast about this and he said, "My God, we always have to use home visits. We can't effect any change without them." But skilled teaching isn't a priority. The priority is to help these kids eliminate some of their sort of more grossly acted-out behavior problems.

I think of Eddie, for example. This is a small child with Down's syndrome who used to spit at his father. It's one of those behaviors that the parent unconsciously reinforces in the child when he's little, and then when he starts getting older, the parent doesn't think it's cute any more. It follows a typical kind of treatment pattern where it gets worse before it gets better. If he's doing it pretentiously, that is, when father started ignoring him, his behavior got worse instead of getting better. But again, when you have phenomenon like this, it's very helpful to have a group leader or a home visitor say to the father, "Hang in there—keep it up; this is a predictable phenomenon; this is going to happen. If you hang in there the behavior will go away in five or six weeks." And it does. It's much harder to say that in a manual for behavioral change. It might be that a manual accompanied by a record, which simply repeats what the book says, or a filmstrip or video cassette might possibly package behavior management in the home equally well, but, at the moment, some evidence that we're beginning to get says that in terms of skilled teaching, you can do as well if not better through a packaged kind of media approach. When it comes to behavior management possibly that's where the professional should get some inputs.

We combined our various outcome measures (i.e., changed behavior) did multiple regressions of 27 demographic background characteristics to see what would be predictors of how well families would do. And we did an overall predictor, so that in pulling all of our treatment conditions together, we got a multiple R of 0.4, which explained about 16 percent of the variance and was terribly unexciting. We then repeated it, condition by condition, and got multiple R's in the range of 0.87 to 0.92, which are incredibly high. This means that effectively given a whole series of background characteristics which we could get in a paper and pencil test before anyone ever began training, we could predict about 80 percent of the variance as to how well they were going to do, given the training condition they were in.

Some of my colleagues feel that was lucky and that if we try to replicate, we would probably come up with entirely different results. They may very well be right, but there are some things within the predictor equations that seem to make a great deal of sense. For example, in the manuals-only condition, the families that did best— facilitators in that condition—were families where the mother's education and the family's socioeconomic status was high. These people are going to be on their own, and they're going to have to make use of the manuals with no one to interpret them. An inhibitor in that condition would be other siblings or children in the home. In a group-plus-visit condition, however, other kids in the home turn out to be a facilitator. The reason is that our in-home visitors consciously brought the siblings in as treatment agents. For the last three years, we've been running a large-scale program to train brothers and sisters of retarded children to accept the problems and live with their retarded siblings. So that, for instance, a family with many brothers and sisters is an inhibitor in manuals only, but it could be a facilitator in group-plus-visit.

Another kind of negative predictor in the group-visit condition is that the parents that participate in other groups, presently or in the past, consistently do more poorly in terms of carrying out programs for their own child. We've always assumed in the past that many of the kind of social-worker-led groups in the mental health field for mothers seemingly didn't do them any good but probably didn't do them much harm. I'm speaking particularly of groups that are geared toward expression of feelings and guilt. It may turn out that a parent who has adjusted to that form of interacting with an agency and her child will have in fact more difficulty or will not see a need to go home and actually teach the child. A group like ours is geared much more toward training people in action. In other words, we do much better with parents who do not have other kinds of group experiences to begin with.

Parental Change through Training Curricula

One of the other areas we looked at was the attitudes, feelings, and opinions that parents had as a result of this training experience. The main kind of attitude change that one gets is that parents seem to feel considerably more capable of evaluating the services their kids are getting than they did before they went through this kind of experience. They have always been very high in terms of their demands for services. We are pleased to see that it didn't get any less. But, they feel more capable of evaluating the outside school services that their child is getting. If one looks, for instance, at countries that have a good continuum of services, such as the Scandinavian countries, one sees that, there, the parents have had the main influence in changing the retardation system. In Scandinavia, one group became very politically active. The head of the group was a lawyer who became the head of retardation in Denmark, and by being very politically active, brought about changes in the kind of service delivery. Now that's happening in the United States, in states that have active parents associations, such as Pennsylvania and Massachusetts. Parents are initiating class action suits and are bringing about a demand for more services.

Thus, what we really need is a more comprehensive system of services for retarded kids, and these training programs are only one little piece along the way toward comprehensiveness. It is an interesting piece, as one of its effects is to make parents more sensitive to the whole system of services. One of the other things that we're interested in doing now is taking these materials and packaging them into a training curriculum for groups such as the National Association for Retarded Citizens, a huge organization with chapters in.every small town across the country.

By and large, parents come together once a month for coffee and talk over new subjects. It could be anything from flower arranging for the retarded to camping to whatever. We're considering putting together a one-year curriculum for the National Association for Retarded Citizens chapters, so people can take manuals, film strips, youth groups, service groups, community groups, etc., and essentially train parents in being able to more effectively deal with their kids at home and hopefully at the same time make a more cohesive force within the associations. We've also been involved fairly centrally in the last year in the use of manuals and training programs to change services in large-scale institutions down to small developmental centers throughout New England.

A Representative Training Program

In fact, I've run an experimental summer camp for retarded and disturbed children for the last five years now. Part of the camp program is a large training grant from the social and rehabilitation services to do behavioral training of institutional staff throughout New England. We're really limited in terms of what our training can be, because the model is to bring people to camp for perhaps a week or two, have them live in, and in a combination of seminars, actually do stuff with kids while they're on-site so they're able to go back and change the settings. What happens is the people become a little more proficient in dealing with kids, but they don't become very much more proficient in terms of setting-change problems.

So what we've done over the years is to develop a program where we try to teach the most of the procedures before and after camp with a series of instructional manuals, and we spend the time at camp with a vertical cross-section of the administrative hierarchy. We use time during the week to plan ways in which they're going to change the settings when they go back home. Thus, in order for a group to come to camp, an organization must send us a vertical cross-section of their staff. It must consist of at least four people. It might be the director, then the director of nurses, then two teachers and a teacher's aid, a parent, and then the chairman of their board of directors, for instance.

We take that group to the camp for a week and work with them on developing a specific plan of action for changes in their setting using the manuals to transmit most of the behavioral modification inputs that we used to do through lectures and seminars, etc., so that we don't have to waste time. One of their intervention plans when they return is to do in-service training for their other staff and community training for parents who aren't directly served by them, so that they use the manuals as a vehicle. It makes such an enormous difference for a person who feels uncertain in his own skills to have this manual to use.

Of course, our manuals are just the first step. When you get a whole series of film strips, videotapes, and other kinds of instructional manuals as a resource for people, they're going to be much more brave in setting up a decent in-service education program.

Many of the facilities we deal with are in rural Maine, Vermont, and New Hampshire, where many parents do not get any services. The clinics don't do a lot of outreach in part because they don't really know what to do. They're not really sure how they're going to go into a home and be of any kind of help, and they see their whole thing in terms of how many beds or how many places they have in the classroom there.

An Analysis of the "New Approach"

Across the board, our self-help manuals are the most effective because we spent the most time developing them. We have a series of five at different levels, whereas in speech we have only two, and in play we have only two, and in behavioral problems we have only one. Our behavioral problem manuals are least effective, because that is one area in which you cannot give a prescribed program. What you have to do is teach people a way of looking at a child and figuring out what's going on between them and the child, in his environment. Then coming out of the program you can give them sort of a trouble-shooting list of steps and a way of looking at the child that you can't give them in a program that says, "If the child bangs his head against the wall, if the child is self-stimulating, and if the child kicks his brother—do this, this, and this," because that wouldn't make any sense; whereas, you can do that in some other areas. You can in a play manual show parents how to teach a child to ride a bicycle.

The manuals had an interdisciplinary group of people such as speech therapists, nurse, psychologists, and some special educators and occupational therapy consultants working on them. The programs themselves went through a whole series of development. We even tested some of our initial hypotheses. For instance, we hypothesized that there would not be a very good correlation between a child's level in speech and language his or her level in self-help skills. So that we couldn't have a common basic, intermediate,, and advanced manual because the child that was basic in speech and hearing might be advanced in self-help. We decided we needed specific manuals for different areas, but we further assumed, and this was true, that within a given area like self-help, there would be a high correlation between various self-help skills. That kids that were higher in grooming would also be high in dressing. If true, this meant that we could get away with putting various skills within the same area.

We did empirical tests of that within state institutions and within families. These tests were simply skill assessment and looking at the interrelations between child levels, so that we could decide empirically where the cut-off should be for the various manuals and which specific skills were apt to be scattered, and therefore, should be put in several manuals. Some skills can be scaled better than other skills. So we did a whole series of pilot tests both on the materials that go into the manuals and then a whole series of testing involving parents. It's hard for parents to critique materials because they haven't got anything to compare them to. They're so gratified to get anything that they are very pleased. We started giving parents our manuals plus a series of other things that are being developed for parents. We also gave parents comparisons between ours and other materials and questionnaires that asked a lot of specific questions that began to give us some insight into how to change things.

One of our biggest difficulties was finding illustrations that were acceptable to parents of the retarded. Children who look normal in appearance; they don't look like kids that many of these folks have. If they look too straight, they're not fun; if they look too humorous, you might be making fun. We got a lot of feedback from parents and families on this. We did about 15 mini-test studies along the way. We did studies with rural populations in Maine and in the Indian reservations in South Dakota just on terms of reading level and whether people could read these things because we didn't make an intentional effort to write it at a third- or fourth-grade level. We wrote it the way we speak and we said how many people are going to lose as a result of that? And in fact we're finding out that you lose quite a few people on the reservation in South Dakota and that there's now an effort out there to translate the materials into a more straightforward language.

In conclusion, let me suggest that the biggest thing that could have been done for mentally retarded people would have been to have actualized the war on poverty, because that would have wiped out about 80 percent of the retarded. One of the ways that the retardation problem is being attacked now, in a different way, is the number of these class action suits and new state legislation about rights to education, because many of the kids that are labeled retarded are because the schools don't want to deal with them. They may be Spanish-speaking or they may be black kids who act out. They are given an I.Q. test and called retarded and put in a special class, whereas three other kids in class who would have also tested out at I.Q. 75 rarely get labeled because they don't cause a problem that gets them tested in the first place.

Jane Mercer, a sociologist, has written a book called *Labelling the Mentally Retarded* (1973). She's done some large-scale studies of the process by which certain people get that label. A lot of people have become sensitive to that and there's now new legislation on the books of some states, including a very progressive law in Massachusetts, which as yet has no funding to enforce it. Chapter 766 of the Massachusetts code in effect does away with all diagnostic labels of kids and talks about the right of every child from 3 to 21 to have an education and obligates the state to pay for that education up to whatever it costs. It's got a great deal of parent involvement and a parent appeal process, so that the child cannot be labeled retarded and put into a special trap without the parent having a whole series of appeals. That, in and of itself, is going to begin to make a big change since many children aren't going to get the label.

We should not do what we've done in the past, create a lot of specific kinds of retardation-creating environments such as state schools, which take the child and make him progressively more retarded, so he comes out as a very nonfunctioning adult. Simply keeping people out of institutions and providing the whole series of community programs that are beginning to get filled in, such as preschool education for parents, reschool nurseries, therapeutic summer camps, sheltered workshops, prevocational training programs, vocational training programs beginning in late adolescence, etc., can give many people that are functioning at a fairly retarded level (I'm talking about organic cases, IQ's below 50, specific diagnoses such as Down's syndrome) opportunities there they *can* function, *can* live in a community, *can* live at least semi-independently, *can* function in either competitive employment in fairly menial jobs or in sheltered kinds of employment. This is in contrast to paying $13,000 a year like it costs Rhode Island to keep people who could be self-supporting in an institution. No one knows the limits to how far people can be pushed. The group of children like the ones I'm dealing with now were called severely retarded 10 years ago. Now it's true that many of the kids I'm dealing with are going to have to live still in a somewhat sheltered environment the rest of their lives, but a lot them aren't.

One of the reasons children do badly on I.Q. tests is that the retarded have a whole series of learning experiences that are failures. So an I.Q. test is a new chance to fail, and many people have documented that the retarded develop a strategy of approaching a task which is failure-avoiding, rather than success-seeking. This means that very often their responses are such that they end up looking very retarded because they're just trying to get the situation over with.

I.Q. tests measure such things as attention, how well someone can quickly relate to a stranger and measures a very limited range of cognitive skills. Many of the questions on the test are completely beyond the experience of a kid who's grown up in an institution. Also, there are a lot of things you can do with a retarded child to raise I.Q. I've gotten dramatic I.Q. changes with children at camp. You can teach them a lot of the underlying processes that they need to take I.Q. tests. In fact, one of the things that we often do is teach them how to take I.Q. tests.

Of course the question arises, aren't we just changing the label, but not necessarily changing the condition? That's right, but at least it can be standardized. Labeling is different, town by town,, state by state. The child is most apt to get the label when he is in the school system. For a lot of us, the school systems are the only time in life when everybody has to do the same thing and function according to standardized norms. In the schools, for example, of the city of Cambridge, Mass., the I.Q. cutoff point for being labeled a slow learner is 79. If you're in the city of Boston, it's 75, but if you're somewhere else it might be 85. A student who was tested in Newton, Mass., a wealthy suburb of Boston, was called retarded with an I.Q. of 120. They say this child is slow, he's not hanging in; well that's because his class is very high, you know, and he's 120. So it's terrifically relative.

There's fifteen times as many retarded people per capita in Washington, D.C. as in Alabama. Why is that? It's because Alabama doesn't have any services, so there's no point in labeling someone if it doesn't mean anything. Discrimination is based on observed difference that's meaningful in a given context. So, it's a funny kind of social problem and it cuts across a lot of areas.

If you're interested in the effect of physical environment and architecture, all you have to do is spend a day in a state institution and see how you function when you get home. The whole of that environment says act in a strange, animal like way: Don't look out the window, because the windows are up there, and they have bars on them. You must be somebody that's dangerous, because the lights all have grids over them. you must be sort of like an animal, because the floor has a drain in the middle of it. you must have something medically wrong with you, because the staff is wearing white uniforms. You know, by the time a kid finishes a day in an institution, what's left? And in fact, a lot of the new settings that are being built are still that way. There's so many constituencies in an institution that have power, like the nursing service. The federal state school is the oldest school for the retarded in the country, and it's the one I've worked in for years. I used to direct a children's unit there. That's another story, but they developed the whole series into cottages. Each cottage has a nursing station in it, because the nurses insisted upon that.

There are many people interested in environmental relationships that could talk about the development of community residences and alternatives. Some of the different things you find are group foster care, the predominant model in California and in Vermont; small group homes, family-style group homes, where the maximum would be about 10 children and 10 adults . We're talking about adults now; the medium-sized group homes from about 11 to 20; and what we've called large group homes from 20 to 50 which have very different manifestations of programming because of different staff patterns in homes of different sizes, so in that dimension size is important. A group of places that we call mini-institutions that have 50 to a 100 people in them consider themselves group homes in the community, but by virtue of their size have to be different in terms of the quality of life.

There are sheltered villages, where the orientation is not at all to integrate the retarded person into the community, but to create an independent community. There are also homes for the elderly, which are mixed group homes where mentally ill and retarded people are put together. Semi-independent living arrangements are defined in Massachusetts as any kind of setting for the retarded where there's not a full-time staff. Boarding houses are a very interesting kind of process to develop because they can be made self-supporting. They sometimes just need a little help to get started. Workshop dormitories, where people live and work in the same facility are also outlawed in Massachusetts by administrative guidelines.

In Massachusetts, in order to start a group home, people must be working in a separate place. In Pennsylvania, for instance, there are workshop dormitories where people live and work under the same roof. They're the single best model in terms of turnover, getting people through and into the community, because there's a real integration between how people are working and what they're doing in the house.

Nursing homes are the main vehicle now for moving people out of state institutions. And even within those, there's an enormous variety in the kind of philosophy. For instance, we visited a sheltered village where retired nuns are living with retarded people. Kind of a quiet place. It's slow. We visited one that's anthroposophic, in which a group of German intellectuals that have moved to the United States set up a place where they live with the retarded; a very interesting kind of place. I don't know a lot about it, but according to some of my staff who visited it, it's clearly got a philosophical base in terms of the life here and now and its relation to the life after. Because of their expense sheltered villages tend to have very wealthy people in them.

There is a whole series of other settings, but the point is that every state I've mentioned, because of the particular interests of the people at power in that state, has picked a model to subscribe to. There are clear exceptions. Nebraska has a network of services. Pittsburgh has an interesting large private organization called Transitional Services, which gives a whole variety of experiences and does some very interesting things. Most of the group home movement is based upon middle- class philosophies and neighborhoods. They are not found in the hard core of large urban areas. The people in Pittsburgh say, "Well, hell, you know, that's where many of these people came from, that's where many of them are going to have to live if they take basic menial jobs like custodians," etc. So they've moved into areas that, by and large, are areas that are not high crime areas, that are more like university areas, but are still kind of run-down. Large group homes essentially teach many of the people to live off welfare; in other words, some group home sponsors don't feel that they have to train everybody to have a job. I mentioned that the other night at a meeting in Rhode Island and many well meaning group home advocates became very angry and nearly got thrown out of the place. I don't subscribe to it necessarily, but that's what is happening in many places.

If you have consistent difficulty getting along with your peers and worry a lot about getting ahead with your work, are you ever so slightly mentally or emotionally ill and in need of treatment? Or are you simply lacking some skills of perceiving others, judging yourself, and influencing other people's reactions to you? Bernard Guerney describes three ways of accounting for emotional and behavioral problems and develops a clear distinction between such problems, where they are seen as afflictions needing medicine and where they are seen as psychological learning problems. Guerney describes the role of a new kind of human development specialist which he calls the psychosocial educator and shows how the roles of this person can replace what in old fashioned medical model speech is called prevention, diagnosis and treatment. He also argues that among other virtues of the psychosocial educator is that the client is more likely to be treated with, and then to learn of his own, dignity and respect.

Chapter 17

THE DELIVERY OF MENTAL HEALTH SERVICES: SPIRITUAL VS. MEDICAL VS. EDUCATIONAL MODELS

Bernard Guerney, Jr.

When I speak to a group of students on these models of mental health services delivery, the first thing I usually do is conduct a survey. I say to the group, "Like everyone else, there are aspects of the way you function as people about which you are dissatisfied: you have certain habits, you have certain ways that you relate to other people, or fail to relate to other people, that cause you to feel dissatisfied with yourself. There are certain aspects of your behavior that you believe are not pleasing to important people in your life, which you would like to alter if you could. There are ways in which you deal with your emotions that you would like to change, or ways in which you deal with your work or with other people that you would like to improve. I'm sure you have such personal problems."

I tell them to pick a problem along these lines that is most disturbing to them. I then say, "With that problem in mind, I'd like you to tell me what you think has caused that problem and the source of assistance you would prefer if you were to seek help in overcoming that problem." I say I will present them with three alternative views dealing with the cause and remedy of their problem. To assure anonymity, I tell the group to close their eyes and to rest their heads down on the table or arm of the chair and from this position to raise their hands when I mention an alternative which they think applies to them and their problem. I assure them I will pay no attention to them as individuals in registering their replies, that I am interested only in the general tally and thus that they need have no fear of embarrassing themselves in any way.

The first of the alternatives is, "How many of you believe that your problem is due to some kind of supernatural force—some kind of possession by bad spirits or the devil—and that to get help with this problem you should go to someone who could get rid of the bad spirits or exorcise the devil?" In a class of about 35, usually only one or two will raise their hands.

The second question I ask is, "How many of you think your difficulty is a sort of sickness or a neurotic condition and that medical or psychiatric assistance is the kind of help you should seek if you want help?" Generally, four or five students raise their hands.

I then present the third and final possibility: "How many of you think that your difficulties are based on ways that you have learned to handle your emotions, ways that you've learned to react to other people or come to expect others to react to you, and that you should seek the help of someone who could teach you to handle your emotions differently or revise your behavior or your expectations about the behaviors of others?" Generally, except for two or three people who haven't raised their hands for any of the options, the remainder of the class raise their hands for this alternative.

The Spirit Model

The first alternative, the spirit model, represents the model for viewing and treating mental and emotional prolems that was prominent until the late nineteenth and early twentieth century. It is now clearly less prominent, but by no means extinct. In a recent popular survey, something like 48 percent of those questioned said that they believe in the devil. Perhaps the recent popularity of the film, *The Exorcist*, influenced these results. But it is also possible that belief in the devil had something to do with the popularity of the film.

The attraction of the spirit theory still is strong enough to influence many people, even in the realm of common physical ailments. Less than a week ago, I watched a television show claiming to be scientific in which a highly educated American suffering from bursitis went to an African Witch Doctor who used a chicken to draw out evil spirits from the patient. The Witch Doctor then killed the chicken, thereby, the patient claimed, curing him of bursitis. If you think in worldwide terms, rather than only in terms of highly industrialized nations, the devil and his fellow spirits are alive and well when it comes to people's conceptions of emotional and interpersonal problems. On a more everyday level, many people, including a fair number of otherwise intelligent and educated individuals, take at least some guidance in conducting their personal and interpersonal affairs from astrology, which is not exactly part of the Spirit Model, but it's within the same realm. Nevertheless, my little classroom surveys suggest that among the highly educated, the Spirit Model is clearly *not* the prevailing model among our educated youth.

The Medical Model

The second model, the medical model, is the model which came into dominance in this century and which is the dominant model today insofar as the organization and delivery of mental health services is concerned. It represents a great improvement, of course, over the Spirit Model. Helping people no longer had to involve such things as trephination to let the spirits out or using sticks literally to beat the devil out of them. The stigma of being mentally ill may be less than the stigma of being possessed by the devil; it is nevertheless very strong. And, as my survey shows, the medical model does not represent the way most highly educated people—and I'd venture to say the majority of less educated people as well—tend to view their own problems; nor does it reflect their preferences about sources of help for emotional and interpersonal problems. It seems to have only a little more appeal than the spirit model.

How then did the medical model gain such a predominant place in our conceptions of emotional and interpersonal problems, and gain such a firm grip on the resources and methods for providing the public with service?

The Rise of the Medical Model

A major factor, of course, is that the medical model *is* an appropriate model for dealing with many problems that plague people in terms of their emotional functioning, particularly those problems which are acute and severe. There is a strong interaction between genetic predispositions, biochemistry, and enviromental factors in determining what we learn about handling our emotions and behaviors.

Deficiencies in certain biochemical substances, such as vitamins for example, will lead to emotional disturbances. The introduction of even the most minute quantities of certain chemicals, for example, LSD, can have extreme effects on our moods and our emotional functioning. Studying the interplay of these factors clearly involves the medical model in an extremely important way. And the manipulation of biochemistry—adding, subtracting and neutralizing various biochemical substances in our bodies by physical means—no doubt will, and should, continue to play a vital role in helping people to function better emotionally. The only thing under question here is the application of the medical model where no physical disabilities or physical treatments are involved.

The second factor to consider in understanding the predominance of the medical model is that medicine experienced a sharp rise in its ability to help cure physical ailments during this century. Its broad extension into behavioral realms was an inevitable by-product of the great benefits to mankind it was continuously demonstrating.

Third, the early theorists who dealt with emotional and interpersonal difficulties were physicians. It was natural for them to think of such problems in terms of analogies to physical disease, (traumas, symptoms, etc.) and medical practice (sickness, treatment, cure, etc.). The theories based on these analogies were quite convincing, and the terminology stuck so fast as to make it difficult to think of the process of helping people in any other terms but those of medical practice.

Fourth, there was and is the factor of political dominance. Physicians controlled the major institutions which were in a position to provide services to people in need of help. Since there is the psychosomatic factor we spoke of earlier—the interaction between the realms of learning and behavior on the one hand, and genetics and biochemistry on the other—it was probably inevitable that the institutions that dispensed physical help would come to be the dispensers of psychological help. They were serving the public and in control of the institutions providing service for a long time before behavioral scientists emerged from the universities to apply their special knowledge of psychological environments, the learning process, and the laws governing behavior, to the problems which individuals had in struggling to cope with their emotions and with other people. When the behavioral scientists and their students came out into the "real" world, all the positions of institutional power were already firmly occupied. The influences of institutional dispensations and sanctions can be almost as powerful in influencing professionals as anyone else. But I believe that more subtle factors were even more important: it is natural for those out of power to look to those in power for guidelines as to what is and is not the proper way to think about and solve problems.

Those of you who have had some comparative psychology know about the phenomenon of *imprinting*. For example, there's a certain stage in the very early life of a duckling when it will establish a long-lasting pattern of behaving toward whatever kind of animal happens to be present in that critical formative period as if that animal were its mother. If it was a dog that was present, the duckling would follow the dog around for a long period afterwards as if it were the mother duck. When the behavioral scientists emerged after World War II, they entered almost exclusively into medical facilities. The mother-person, or, if you prefer, the father-figure, was always the physician. For their whole infancy and early adulthood as professionals, psychologists and other behavioral scientists have been following a pseudo-mother. Yet behavioral practitioners are not physicians, and most important, they *do* have true mothers and fathers—scientists and educators in the universities.

The Decline of the Medical Model

In the past 15 years or so, thanks largely to the efforts of adherents to the teachings of Carl Rogers and B. F. Skinner, more and more providers of psychological services are abandoning one major component of the medical model. They are abandoning the *disease* conception and the illness analogies, in the way they approach those great numbers of people who seem to have problems in living that are not primarily biochemical in nature.

The new breed has adopted learning theory in place of disease conceptions, and a new terminology is beginning to replace medically derived terminology. The new terminology is one that is more suitable for the large numbers of people who need psychological help but are not mentally ill, i.e. not biochemically imbalanced or organically deficient. But the new breed has not yet abandoned another crucial aspect of the medical model. Even the behaviorists, for example, have suffered severe culture lag in this respect. The medical model still serves as a paradigm for the *delivery* of mental health services. It is still based on the model provided by the practitioner of medicine, the physician, rather than on the practitioner of education, the teacher. Those offering psychosocial help still conceive of themselves and certainly act as, *clinicians* and not as psychosocial *educators*. As long as this remains true, we will never be able to meet the great need for ameliorative, let alone preventative, psychosocial services. Unless the practitioner sees clearly the different implications and consequences of adapting one or the other of these two role models, progress will be retarded.

Old models of practice don't die, and they don't fade away, until a more viable model can be perceived. Despite the fact that it has been in fashion for decades to speak of psychotherapy as an educational process and to attempt to explain it in terms of learning theory, a vital step remains to be taken: the development of a system for delivering services based on the model developed by educators. Yet I firmly believe that the way in which the educator delivers services to the public provides a model far superior to the way of the physician when it comes to psychological services.

The United States, indeed the world, is suffering from mass psychosocial illiteracy. The behaviors of individuals in families and in our places of work (and, yes, in education) are producing emotional casualties far faster than traditional methods of service can rehabilitate them. Without a change in the delivery system that will provide more effective and more durable help and, above all, problem prevention, we, as providers of psychosocial services, will continue to fail. The model provided by practitioners of mass education offers us a way out of our Sisyphean predicament. Not only does the educational model recommend itself upon analysis, but also, as revealed by our informal survey, the public appears to be ready and waiting for its ascendance: it is viewed as the most suitable model by the highly educated public and, we suspect, the poorly educated as well.

The Educational Model

I find that when I talk about the educational model, students often equate it with the behavior modification movement and equate the psychoeducator with the behavior therapist. This is not at all my view. The educational model of service delivery can be employed to implement many different theoretical orientations. Some orientations, of course, lend themselves to it more readily than others; but I can think of no theoretical position that it would not serve. It can encompass the Freudian along with the Skinnerian. A case can even be made that Freud was the godfather of the movement since he made the first, albeit primitive, use of the educational model in treating little Hans by training the boy's father to work with Hans rather than doing it himself. It is not Freud's fault that his more devout disciples failed to follow him in this particular giant step while they followed so many others.

Although the practicing psychosocial educator had his historical roots in the educational system to begin with, his return to the educational model would not represent a step backward. It is more like a person returning to his hometown after having been around the world—in this case the world of people's emotional and interpersonal troubles and aspirations—and who now seeks to combine his old knowledge with his new knowledge. Everything he has learned in working with emotionally troubled clients should be employed in implementing his new educational programs. Therefore, the psychosocial educator would be a far cry from the traditional educator in many ways.

The settings in which the psychosocial educator would function would not be limited to formal scholastic institutions. I hope he will be able to win a secure place in formal scholastic settings from kindergarten through graduate school, both in departments of student services and as a teacher of a new part of the regular curriculum. But his arena of operations should certainly extend beyond the formal system of schooling: it would extend into community mental health centers, guidance clinics, industrial settings and new types of educational institutions—schools for training in everyday living—which he himself would design and administer.

What he teaches would, of course, be very different than the kinds of things currently taught in educational settings. His objectives would not be to increase intellectual understanding as such, but rather would be the objectives sought by psychotherapists: increasing emotional and interpersonal competencies and life satisfactions. The main criteria of his success would not be changes in intellectual understanding, although that would be involved, but the increased personal satisfaction his students can derive from new attitudes toward themselves and others, and new competency and flexibility in the way they deal with their physical environment, their emotions, their behavior, and their relationships with others.

Programs aimed at increasing satisfaction might include, for example, learning how to become more (or less) cooperative with others, more (or less) sexually inhibited, or more (or less) fearful of physical dangers. Husbands, wives, parents and children might take courses teaching them how to develop less conflicted, more harmonious, and more intimate relationships. We hope that it will prove possible to develop an educational program for every type of emotional problem now treated by traditional psychotherapeutic methods.

The educator, whatever his orientation, would teach the probable consequences of various types of behaviors, in various types of situations with different types of people, and would make known the value judgments implicit in various behavioral choices. But above all, he will be interested in increasing *skills*, in increasing the behavioral repertoire and behavioral flexibility of his students, in teaching people to be able to behave as they wish to behave in given situations. Like teachers of music, auto repair, or pottery, he will deal in "how to do it." Unlike them, however, the skills he would teach would not involve relatively impersonal objectives and tangible objects, but emotions, people, and content that are very close to the core of the student's self-concept, ego, superego and defense mechanisms.

This new kind of educator would incorporate psychotherapeutic methods in his teaching and would be attuned to the subtleties of conflicting motivations and ambivalent feelings, the difficulty of crossing the gap between knowing and doing, the importance of reinforcement, of the self-concept and of interpersonal relationships in trying to teach people how to change themselves and those around them. The incorporation of such knowledge into his teaching methods would make the psychosocial educator a *better* teacher, not something *other* than a teacher.

To summarize, the psychosocial educator's work would be to *teach personal and interpersonal attitudes, concepts, and skills which the individual can apply presently and in the future to solve psychosocial problems and to enhance his and others' accomplishments and satisfactions.*

It is fashionable today to refer to certain psychotherapeutic practices within the medical model as "educational." Hence I would like to spell out some of differences in the two modes of practice. There are not absolute differences, of course, but differences in attitudes, orientation, and emphases.

Differing Emphases in the Medical vs. the Educational Model

Clinical vs. Programmatic Efforts

The clinical practitioner following the medical model tends to think in terms of one person at a time. To him, each individual must be analyzed individually before he feels free to proceed with the helping process. He tends to take each person as he comes and fashion a treatment program for that individual without giving much thought to commonalities among the people he helps and how those commalities might be considered in fashioning more effective and efficient treatment plans.

The practitioner who follows an educational model tends to think in terms of large numbers and in terms of common everyday psychosocial needs and problems that many individuals share. He then can design systematic training programs whereby many others could be trained in skills that would help them to solve their problems or meet their psychosocial goals. Priorities in developing such programs can be set in terms of depth and/or scope of needs and problems, but eventually the goal would be to meet all the needs now being met by practitioners following the medical model. The psychosocial educator believes that by being programatic, he can, so to speak teach fire-fighting and fire prevention skills to many and therefore realistically hope to save many lives; whereas, if he himself ran around putting out one fire after another, he could save only a small number.

Diagnostic vs. Goal Orientation

The clinical practitioner tends to think in terms of needing to locate pathology and design his individual prescriptive program to eliminate pathology. The psychosocial educator tends to think in terms of the aspirations and desires of his client and wishes to teach him how to reach them. Even when the client starts with a complaint or something he wants remedied, it should be possible to translate the negative objective into a positive one, making it feasible to embark upon skill-training, the building in of enduring strengths and skills, rather than only the removal of an irritation or weakness.

Individual vs. Group Methods

The differentiation here is not as sharp as in the previous illustrations. The advent of group psychotherapy has changed things somewhat; nevertheless, the clinical practitioner following the medical model not only does his thinking and planning in terms of individuals, but usually administers his treatment to one person at a time. The psychosocial educator knows that at one time individual tutoring was all the educational model had to offer, and that some individual tutoring will probably always be a part of his procedures for practical reasons, especially when the caseload is a small one. Nevertheless, wherever possible and practical, he tends to think of groups as being the most appropriate and efficient units for instruction. He is interested in employing every kind of economical and efficient aid which is practical and realistic, from specially trained teaching assistants to programmed texts, films, and videotapes.

Insular vs. Outreaching Methods

The traditional mental health practitioner, following the model of the physician and many other professionals, waits in his office for individuals to find him, usually by way of a referral from some other professional person. The psychosocial educator would run scheduled programs and must often use public media to let the public know that a particular program is currrently open to enrollment. In the manner of business schools and adult education programs, it is desirable, in fact necessary, for him to announce his offerings, in factual and dignified terms, and to as broad a segment of the public as he can reach.

Closed vs. Shared Planning

The clinical practitioner generally does not share the outcomes of his tests and measures in a detailed way with his clients, giving them the vital statistics and probabilities associated with various tests and procedures. He usually keeps these things to himself and presents only his own conclusions to the clients. What psychotherapy client has been privy to information about the validity, or lack of proven validity, with respect to a Rorschach or TAT test he has taken? The psychosocial educator, on the other hand, typically gives all such information and probabilities to those seeking his guidance. With such information and sharing in the thought processes and deliberations of the counselor, the client typically makes his own choices. The client being evaluated for traditional psychotherapy is more typically in the position of being told in effect that he either "needs" it, or he doesn't "need" it. Very often the potential therapist himself is not aware of how much his decisions are based on sheer value judgments which he has come to think of not as products of his own subculture and professional training, but as matters of "sickness" and "health," or "maladjustment." The psychosocial educator is in a much better position to recognize that the client himself should have the right to select the behaviors he wishes to strengthen or diminish, and that such choices are largely a matter of value judgment.

The expanded use of the educational model should also permit the development of tests of aptitude and achievement that will allow the psychosocial educator to use testing and counseling procedures more akin to that of the educational counselor than they are to the procedures of the present-day psychodiagnostician. When this improvement in specificity and validity of psychological testing comes to pass, the psychosocial educator cannot only be open about his value judgments and ask the client to examine his values in making his decisions, but he should be in a position to make reasonably accurate predictions about how much a particular client will benefit from taking one kind of educational program as compared to another. There would be no reason for him not to share all such information openly with the client.

Exclusive vs. Open Contracts

I am not referring here to any formal contractual arrangements, but rather to implicit contracts, sets of mutual expectations which characterize physician–patient relationships on the one hand, and educator–student relationships on the other. Within his area of specialization, the physician expects the client to be under his exclusive care, and he expects to decide if any other professional should be. The public has been inculcated in this expectation and violates it only rarely, semicovertly, and with trepidation. This expectation is even more true with respect to psychotherapists following the physician's model than it is with physicians per se. It would be quite unusual for a traditional therapist to tell a client that in addition to seeing him, he also ought to be seeing another therapist on a regular basis. The traditional therapists' "patients" understand that to do so would be a grave affront to therapist, muddying the healing waters in some mysterious and dreadful way.

Teachers, on the other hand, usually are eager to see their pupils get as much exposure to the courses of other teachers as they can fit into their schedule. A teacher of German is not at all upset by the notion that a student may also be studying French with another teacher, or even uses a second instructor to speed his learning of German. If I were teaching a program entitled "Increasing Cooperative Behavior," I would not be upset by the fact that a student in this program was also studying "Ejaculation-Control" from another teacher, nor "How to be a More Forceful Competitor," nor even if he were simultaneously taking a second course in "Increasing Cooperative Behavior" from another teacher. It is always understood by educators that information and skill is to be used at the discretion of the learner and that he will use or not use the skills he acquires according to circumstances and his own preferences of the moment. To a teacher, there's no reason to fear a person having too much knowledge, too many skills, or as many teachers as he wants. If the teachers have different methods, so much the better. If they are saying conflicting things, that only opens the way for a student to become a *better* student by asking each teacher more challenging questions and to make his own decisions.

Problem Solving vs. Skill Instruction

Physicians know that ultimately the body must heal itself. Psychotherapists following the physician's image know that ultimately the patient must take responsibility for curing himself and are very quick to say so. Nevertheless, the clinical practitioner obviously sees his *major* role as that of intervening directly to cure illness, not that of teaching people how to understand and deal with their bodies in such a way as to prevent disease and to minister to their illnesses themselves in a knowledgeable way so as to reduce their dependence upon him to the lowest feasible level. Similarly, the psychotherapist uses his own expertise to try to solve his client's problem. He is primarily interested in ridding the patient of a disability.

The educator's line of march, by contrast, is *not* primarily to use his *own* knowledge, insights, and skills to achieve a solution to the problem. He believes that in the long run, and usually even in the short run, the best way to achieve problem resolution is to give the student the knowledge and skills he needs to achieve problem resolution *himself*. He believes that under those conditions, the client will achieve the most realistic and the most durable resolution to his problem. Teachers do not believe in doing the student's homework for him, and they wish their students to acquire sufficient skill to function independently once they complete the training. The goal of the psychosocial educator is to provide the client with the skills he needs to resolve present and future problems himself, skills which will allow him to prevent problems from arising again, and skills which will allow the client to accomplish his own social and emotional objectives.

Potential Advantages of the Educational Model

I won't attempt to cover all the advantages that the mental health movement could derive from the broad scale application of the educational model, but the following are some of the major ones.

Clarification of the Role of Value Judgments in the Helping Process

The implicit contract of "I am sick/"I will cure you" that prevails between those who are seeking and those who are receiving psychological services, and which was copied from the physician–patient contract, has served to obscure the view that both the helper and his client make *choices* of what is desirable. The physician, except when it comes to issues such as abortion and euthanasia, seldom needs to concern himself with value judgments, because the abhorrence of death and physical pain come fairly close to being universally held values. The good psychosocial educator, on the other hand, must be aware of value issues when he designs his courses and should be prepared to make these issues clear to his students, because when teacher-student attitudes and "contracts" replace healing "contracts" and attitudes, the students may well raise the appropriate questions; even if they don't, the educator's credo says they have a right to know.

More Effective Psychotherapeutic Intervention

Nonmedicinal traditional psychotherapy has not established a strong record in terms of scientific evidence of effectiveness. I can't elaborate here on my reasons for believing it, but I do strongly believe that, in comparison, the educational model will provide faster, more effective, and more durable methods of helping people who do not require physical treatment for their emotional difficulties. Even in its infancy, it is beginning to demonstrate its efficiency and effectiveness and to demonstrate this not just clinically, but in terms of scientifically acceptable standards of proof.

An Increased Capacity for Offering Service

The preparation of systematic programs opens the way to providing more service at lower cost for a number of reasons. With systematic teaching programs, it becomes feasible to use texts, programmed learning, films, videotapes, etc. Systematic education aimed at teaching specific emotional and interpersonal skills also permits—analogous to the use of paraprofessionals in the public schools and graduate assistants in the universities—the use of volunteers and paid paraprofessionals to assist the professional. Such paraprofessionals can become as skilled or more skilled in running certain specific psychoeducational programs. The professional can then function mainly as a supervisor, a program designer, and a program evaluator. One of the reasons mental health service is so expensive, and therefore so inadequate to the task of providing help equal to the need for it, is that it has failed to make good use of mass-produced materials and technicians. Without the development of highly specific programmatic treatment programs that can be quality controlled, the use of paraprofessionals is not only inefficient and lacking in direction, it can be dangerous.

Greater Acceptance and Utilization of Services

As my informal survey demonstrated, the public does not like to think of their emotional and social problems in terms of abnormality, illness, neurosis, etc. They prefer to think of getting help in terms of meeting their own goals by means of learning how to do things they want to do. By adopting an educational model, the provider of psychosocial services might find all ages and classes of people more willing to avail themselves of mental health services, and he will certainly find them less defensive and resistant when they do come for service.

Better Client Guidance and Evaluation Techniques

As I see it, techniques of psychosocial assessment have been floundering for decades in a state of unfulfilled promise. Tests of personal and interpersonal function offer less predictive validity and a less valid basis for helping the *professional* to make decisions than we reasonably could expect, and almost no basis at all for helping the client make informed decisions about what directions he should take to help himself. In contrast, tests developed for vocational and educational guidance and to assess scholastic aptitude and performance are much better in these respects. Why? Because they are geared to more specific behavioral criteria, so that tests can be evaluated and perfected with much greater ease, efficiency, and accuracy. Once psychosocial services are based on the educational model, providing clear-cut objectives and performance criteria linked to each educational program, we can expect a matching revolution to take place in the field of personality assessment, a revolution that would make it far more understandable and useful to the professional and the public alike.

Problem Prevention

Mental health professionals have provided only lip service to the cause of primary prevention. They are not really uninterested in providing such service; they are conceptually self-blinded about how to proceed. Because of the medical model, they had constructed walls in their own minds and could not see how to till the prevention fields. The walls were between "sick" and "well," between "maladjusted" and "adjusted," between "neurotic" and "normal." If a physician treats somebody who isn't sick, he's a quack. Mental health workers were willing to follow a pseudo-mother duck, but they didn't want to quack. They felt comfortable only when they could label the people they worked with as "sick" by one term or another. They were so caught up in diagnostic mumbo jumbo which allowed them to justify their intervention into others' life-styles that they just did not know how to proceed with people who would not label themselves sick or allow the professionals to so label them. So they couldn't really get into the field of prevention in an effective or vigorous way.

In contrast, with the educational model there is no conceptual conflict or difficulty in directing one's efforts simultaneously to those with severe, minor, incipient, and potential problems and those with no problems whatsoever but rather with an ambition to scale to new emotional and interpersonal heights. To design a "preventive" program and another "remedial" program in the same area of interpersonal skill presents no greater conceptual or operational shift than would be required to design, for example, two courses in French, one for language majors and one for nonmajors. You might have to supervise one group more closely, pay more attention to details, and expect to achieve less progress in a given amount of time with one group as compared to the other, but what you teach and the way you teach it remain essentially the same. Very often there would be no reason to design two separate programs; one program would serve well for everyone. Later, some of the students might simply need to reenroll for an advanced course in order to get more supervised experience.

In following the educational model, one does not assume that there are some people who are somehow contaminated, as if they were carrying something contagious, who need to be handled apart from others. If there is to be a division of groups, it would be, as in education, on the basis of such things as starting level, competence, and strength of motivation or ambition.

To exemplify the ease of moving from remedial to preventive programs: In the work of my colleagues and myself, a program called "Filial Therapy," originally designed to help emotionally troubled children by training their parents in the skills used by play therapists, was readily adapted to a less intensive training program to teach any parent similar skills useful in rearing their children. Similarly, a program called "Conjugal Therapy," originally designed to help couples with marital difficulties, was easily adapted into a program for training any married couple, and then into a training program for premarital couples, to help them establish more harmonious, satisfying, and intimate relationships and prevent problems from developing. Now, many groups are run that contain happily married couples alongside desperate couples on the brink of divorce.

Better Mental Health Research

The problems of doing research in traditional psychotherapy or behavior therapy when it is not applied via the educational model are enormous. One usually is limited to a case study (However changed by graphs and numbers, we regard single-subject studies as essentially case studies.); it is difficult, practically and ethically, to assign subjects to control groups or to assign them to alternate treatments while controlling for therapist variables. It is difficult to specify precisely what it is that therapists are doing in order to replicate the study.

The adaptation of the educational model changes all this and makes truly scientific studies of various programs of intervention as readily open to scientific study as are different texts and methods of educational instruction. Large numbers of subjects coming into a program with the same goals in mind are readily available; clients more easily and ethically can be first assigned to alternate programs or asked to wait until the next round of courses, during which time they can serve as controls; and the researcher can specify what is going on in each of the treatment programs with enough specificity so they can be replicated by other investigators.

Thus, here at last is the opportunity to systematically assess and compare methods of helping people by scientific methods on a broad scale. The significance of this, of course, lies not only in advancing scientific knowledge per se, but in the fact that the scientific approach provides the most efficient and effective means of improving our methods and eventually helping more people more economically and more surely.

The Rise of the Educational Model

When I first began to use the educational model in the early 1960s and urged students to adapt it as the method of the future, I had to admit that for any number of reasons it was an approach that might never catch on, a revolution that would never come to pass. But I am far less doubtful today. New programs to systematically teach personal and interpersonal skills are coming out by the dozens.

Today there are programs following the educational model that teach control of weight, alcohol-drinking, anxiety, blood pressure, and aggression. There are programs that teach assertiveness, value clarification, leadership, fair fighting, relaxation, meditation, rational analysis of emotional situations, and self-esteem. There are programs that teach empathic understanding of others, effective communication of one's own desires, negotiation and problem-solving skills to parents, to premarital couples, to the aged, to high school students, and to elementary school students. Programs that systematically teach personal, emotional, and interpersonal skills are coming out at a faster and faster rate.

Today, there are inadequately funded, but very numerous, consultation and education departments in many Community Mental Health Centers. Their function is such as to make it natural for them to employ the education model. As yet they are seen by the medical model establishment as providing services different from psychotherapy—that wall we spoke of earlier prevents the traditionalists from seeing and understanding what is going on under their noses. What will happen if, as we believe will be the case, it becomes evident in terms of who uses these services that the wall between the "neurotic" and the "normal" is an imaginary one? What will happen when research begins to demonstrate that systematic education is the most efficient form of (nonphysiologic) *treatment*? How will the psychotherapy establishment react? My hope and prediction is that they will adopt the educational model, and that they will join in developing and employing new educational programs. If they do, the public will have the kind of help they want and need, and the evolutionary process of spirit-through-medical-to-educational models of delivering mental health services will be completed.

Federalism is caught in the dilemma of needing a central mobilization point for national efforts and change, yet is forced to recognize that problems are as varied as the myriad locales and that those most familiar with specific locales have the best chance of solving their problems. Maintaining the federalist structure means a definite diminution of local and state autonomy. Perhaps the most benign form of the exercise of authority devised by man is evaluation, a process by which the federal government can hold states, regions, and communities accountable, while causing in the evaluation agency itself enormous anguish in the form of searching self-examination. Dr. Charles Windle presents a systematic view of evaluation and lucidly expounds how the National Institute of Mental Health is itself caught up in the web of interaction.

Chapter 18

THE RECORD THUS FAR: DIFFICULTIES, FAILURES AND SUCCESSES IN PROGRAM EVALUATION

Charles Windle

Because I am a believer in truth in advertising and contents labeling, let me tell you explicitly what my values and biases are. I'm a researcher by preference, conviction, and habit. This means that I really do favor truth as the major way to make progress, and I usually prefer it to short-run program advantages.

I want to discuss two serious problems in program evaluation, describe a systems view of program evaluation research, and propose a two-pronged strategy for improving program evaluation research.

Problems of Program Evaluation

One problem with program evaluation is the low credibility when evaluation studies are, or appear to be, designed and disseminated to serve vested interests. James Wilson (1973) of Harvard has been said to have formulated two laws: (1) All policy interventions in social problems produce the intended effect if the research is carried out by those implementing the policy or their friends. (2) No policy interventions in social problems produce the intended effect if the research is carried out by independent third parties, especially those skeptical of the policy.

I'm afraid this is more than casual humor or cynicism. We see these laws invoked seriously. Former Secretary of HEW Casper Weinberger has said in testimony before the Senate Subcommittee on Health that a number of the studies done by HEW to evaluate its programs obviously have been designed to bring out the results that were wanted by the people who ordered them initially. He also said "[Natural] alliances [between people administering programs and the beneficiaries of the programs] do develop, and therefore the reports that come in from the people running the programs are basically designed to support their continuation and their increase in size" (Broder, 1973). Such judgements suggest a serious limitation to program evaluation.

The other problem concerns the extent to which studies remain academic exercises without any application. Buchanan and Wholey (1972), after examining current federal evaluation efforts, found that "increasing amounts of money are being budgeted for evaluation—[but that] the impact of evaluation results on program development and improvement over the last two years has been disappointing when compared with the amount of money and effort that has gone into evaluation."

The long-run result of either of these two problems is a low priority to the use of scientific, rational methods, such as program evaluation, to aid decision making. Improvements in program evaluation methods should focus on these two problems.

A Systems View of Program Evaluation

As a background to understanding program evaluation a system concept is helpful, and is illustrated in Figure 1. The program consists of taxpayers supporting officials who support consumer programs, who, in turn, give feedback as taxpayers to the officials about the nature of the program.

Program evaluation elaborates this system and is usually understood to provide reports on improvement which go to the program administrators and staff. In addition, program evaluation formalizes the relations with consumers by getting systematic feedback from them. Program evaluation may also increase the effectiveness of the program by doing certain things like getting records in better order and making staff more alert to the needs of the consumers. In these functions, program evaluation acts as a part of the service program.

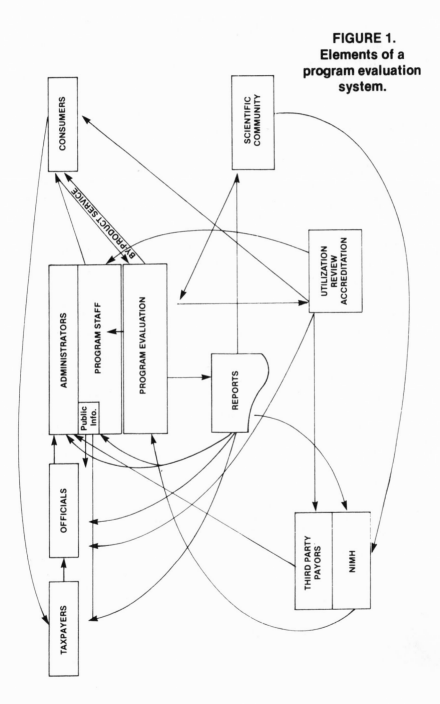

**FIGURE 1.
Elements of a
program evaluation
system.**

Much of the results from evaluations goes directly and informally to the program staff, rather than in a formal end-of-study report. And this is the bane of the researchers. Sometimes in the middle of a study the program staff are convinced that the experimental methods are better and proceed to make changes in the program. The researchers then fail to get data to draw conclusions they consider valid.

A further complication in the system of program evaluation is that researchers also aim their reports to the scientific community. The scientific community rewards program evaluators in professional status and future jobs, which are often in other programs or universities. Ambitious program evaluators are often outward oriented. Thus, they write their reports relatively objectively and according to scientific canons, but underemphasize utility of results by the local program. These reports by outward-oriented researchers tend to be more truthful than reports by other program staff and administrators who have program support as a part of their roles. This distinction in what tends to be reported by different staff is also reflected in an organization's public information activity. Frequently, reports from the program evaluation studies are repackaged by the program staff to better communicate to the program. Such repackaging is likely to be in more intelligible form, but also frequently is substantively more program supportive.

The largest recent innovations in the program evaluation system concern other modes of accountability: utilization review and accreditation. Information about the quality of service programs is required by third-party reimbursement agencies to assure appropriateness of services. Only if utilization review and the accreditation procedures indicate that the particular programs or the services are appropriate will they be reimbursed. These requirements are likely to have a big impact on programs.

A Strategy for Improving Internal Program Evaluation

This strategy applies to the classical form of program evaluation in which a program's own evaluators attempt to improve the program by developing useful information for the staff to use. We've done three things at NIMH in this regard.

Factors in Successful Evalutaions

Two studies examined factors related to success in applied research. Five mental health service research grants were chosen by staff as very successful; and five were chosen as less successful (Glaser and Taylor, 1973). Differentiating factors were sought by visiting the research sites. Successful projects were ones where the researchers had involved the administrators early in the program, whereas the unsuccessful ones did not. Since these were studies of innovative services, and adoption of the innovation was one element of success, it is reasonable that the involvement of the administrator is important.

We found similar results when we looked at program evaluation studies (Windle and Bates, 1974). Our criterion of success was ratings, made soon after the studies were completed, of which studies would be of most and least value relative to their cost. The studies judged most likely to be of value were those in which there had been close collaboration between the contract-researcher and the NIMH staff. Since the NIMH staff were expected to be the primary users, this finding parallels that for research grants.

Literature on Research Utilization

The Human Interaction Research Institute (HIRI) surveyed the literature to identify what factors lead to the utilization of research (NIMH, 1972). There is often a long time lag between when the research was done and when corresponding changes in practice occur. Frequently practitioners lack knowledge available in the scientific literature. And there are often differences in ways of thinking between the researchers and the practitioners.

The HIRI staff have described a number of characteristics of innovations that favor adoption. They also identified organizational characteristics that favor innovation, and communication modes that lead to the adoption of innovations. In general, HIRI's feeling was that ordinary research reports, and even worse, studies in the scientific literature had little value for administrators and practitioners, who seldom read these. Other modes of communication, therefore, are better to use to enhance utilization. Howard Davis of NIMH and HIRI have developed a checklist for change (NIMH, 1972).

As a part of this philosophy, the magazine *Evaluation* is a NIMH-supported attempt to get the ideas about evaluation out to people who might do evaluation. This publication uses a fairly popularized magazine format. NIMH is also supporting conferences on program evaluation, popularizing the need and methods for evaluation. Such approaches seem more socially facilitative of innovation.

NIMH's program evaluation experience

There are still limits on how effective the Davis-HIRI approach is, as we have seen in the program evaluation activities at NIMH. Much of NIMH's program evaluation concerned the Community Mental Health Centers Program, since this program was NIMH's major initiative in mental health services.

This evaluation effort focused on the process of goals of the program, such as continuity, accessibility, responsiveness to needs, and comprehensiveness. For each of these process goals we looked at how successfully were they being attained by the program and under what conditions. Overall, of course, we found that progress was being made by the center's program in these process goals, but that the program was a long way from completely achieving them. We also found some suggestions of ways to facilitate the program (Windle, et al., 1974).

These results are not striking but could be of some help. We found, however, that there was very little utilization of them in any of three different echelons where they might have been used (Windle and Bates, 1974). One echelon is the local community mental health centers. For centers to use the results, they'd have to know the results. Most reports are not widely disseminated nor their availability made widely known. There has been little request for us to disseminate them. Thus, this potential channel of utilization of our program evaluation results has been quite limited.

The second echelon for utilization is NIMH's own program management, which could use results to make program improvements. In fact, it is difficult to find clear examples of such use by NIMH. One reason may be the incompatibility of efforts to improve and efforts to survive. By the time that evaluation results were available, the center's program was under threat by the Nixon administration. It was suggested that the program should be terminated because, since centers had been demonstrated to be successful, there was no need for additional seed-money funding. NIMH had not anticipated so favorable a critique; and the consequence was not what NIMH desired. That result did not stem from our evaluation results; in fact, our results suggested just the opposite, that the program had deficiencies to which more effort needed to be paid. Since program attention was on ways to survive, rather than improve, most of the program evaluation results had little utility.

The third echelon of potential use are superordinate offices, such as the Secretary of HEW and Congress. The results of some of our studies suggest that centers had not fully achieved the seed-money concept of using initial money from the government to build up support from other sources (Harvey, 1970; Marco Systems, 1973). They suggested that the center's program had not really demonstrated its fiscal viability. It was into this dispute concerning whether the center's program had demonstrated its value to the extent of fiscal independence that then Secretary Weinberger came with his claim, cited above, that NIMH's and the Health Services and Mental Health Administration's (HSMHA) evaluation studies were biased and supportive of the program. Obviously, agency program commitments make such bias possible, and led to the choice of this study topic. As a participant in administering these contracts, however, I don't think such biases entered the conduct or reporting of results in these particular studies.

It is clear that we have not perfected the art of utilization of research or instilled it in administrators.

A Strategy for External Program Evaluation

There are a number of new trends that promise other ways in which evaluation may be done. Bert Brown (1973), the director of NIMH, said in 1971 that "the future of mental health and mental retardation is in the area of economics, taxation, and finance." This prediction indicates the major source of the new kinds of program evaluation.

As background it is instructive to look at conditions in the health field, since mental health is closely associated with the health field. A systems analytic report by the HSMHA to Congress in 1972 described weaknesses in the existing health system which, I think, apply to mental health as well (HSMHA, 1972). One was a lack of coordination among provider units, leading to duplication of costly facilities, maldistribution of resources, and lack of continuity of care. Second, legal restrictions on medical practice limit the use of paramedical personnel. Third, an emphasis on fee for service, more insurance for in-patient than alternative forms of care, and full hospital reimbursement encourage more costly care and overprescription of marginally needed services. These things deter care at early stages of illness. Last, "The pervasive influence of the medical profession ... [has made] ... the health system more responsive to the interests of the profession than to the needs of consumers." (HSMHA, 1972) Attempts to solve these problems are producing a number of shifts.

The shifts in financing are somewhat different in the health care and the mental health care systems. In the health system, the shift is from private to public sources of funds. In mental health, there traditionally has been a dual system of state mental hospital service for the poor supported with public funds, and private practitioner outpatient care paid for by people who have enough money. Since 1955, there has been an increase in episodes of care per 100 thousand population in the United States. This increase has been primarily in outpatient clinics and community mental health centers, not state and county hospitals which have declined slightly (Taube & Redick, 1975).

Another measure of trends is the amount of resources that go to different kinds of facilities. Crude estimates are that about 70 percent of mental health expenditures went for state and county mental hospitals in 1956, compared to 57 percent in 1972.

Accompanying these changes are changes in the accountability system. When public money went primarily to state mental hospitals and fees for service were controlled by clients, there was little concern about accountability. As the source of funds changed to third-party payers, concern with appropriateness of care has increased. National health insurance seems a coming trend and is likely to be modeled on the Social Security provisions for monitoring appropriateness and quality of care.

For hospitals to be eligible for Medicare and Medicaid reimbursement, they must have utilization review procedures. These are procedures based upon peer review, usually by physicians, for determining that the care provided in a facility is appropriate. This procedure is motivated primarily to prevent abuses and to contain costs. In order to increase the likelihood that community mental health centers could benefit from this kind of reimbursement, NIMH is encouraging centers to use utilization review.

Utilization review usually is not thought of as a kind of program evaluation, but I believe it should be. It is a less dramatic, continuous form of evaluation based on monitoring, rather than upon direct experiments. But this form of evaluation is highly likely to lead to change in programs. The Social Security amendments now provide incentives for states to establish utilization review by imposing reductions in matching percentages if the Secretary is not satisfied with the state's utilization review procedures.

A second instrumentality for monitoring is the Professional Standards Review Organization (PSRO). The Social Security amendments authorized the establishment of independent PSRO's through which physicians can assume responsibility for reviewing the appropriateness and quality of the services provided under Medicare and Medicaid. This amendment permits the PSROs to utilize the services and accept the findings of utilization review committees in hospitals or other kinds of health care facility, but only to the extent that they're determined to be effective. The review and approval by the PSRO is required as a condition of payment of claims. This provision for PSROs is going to require a monumental effort to develop regulations, standards, procedures, and guidelines. And the care in institutions will have to be reviewed by standards that still have to be developed. There's now a lot of scrambling to try to figure out what can be done. At the start there are likely to be fairly innocuous standards, which may gradually become tightened. Much data are needed about current practice.

A second kind of accountability that is increasing, which I also consider a type of program evaluation, is accountability to the courts. Court rulings such as that in *Wyatt* vs. *Stickney* are establishing that individuals cannot be held involuntarily for treatment if they receive no treatment. It's unclear what criteria the courts can use for judging adequacy of treatment, yet they need to make such determinations.

Gottlieb Simon (1971) sees this issue as undermining the entire rationale for involuntary commitment, which has been the need for treatment. If no treatment is possible this whole rationale collapses. If the state is unwilling to provide treatment or if there's no effective treatment available, a new social policy is desired. Either we will confront our fear and distaste of some social deviants whom we now commit to state hospitals and accept them, or the courts will force us to openly and honestly adopt a policy of preventive detention. This is a program evaluation issue wherein sweeping changes in the care system are possible, and continuous monitoring of the impact of policy is needed, if possible.

The third kind of program evaluation is that of monitoring. NIMH monitor federally funded community mental health centers through site visits, primarily to see that centers comply with regulations. In addition, site visits permit encouragement, guidance, leadership, and information that facilitate change. This site visit procedure is being formalized so that it can be used by states or other interested groups such as citizen bodies.

To assist the monitoring, NIMH collects norms on usual practice in facilities and distributes these both to the facilities, so they can see where they stand compared to other facilities, and to states and regional offices for use in monitoring.

An example is a measure of temporal accessibility of services indicating how many centers provide outpatient care in the evenings as well as the daytime. In 1971 the rate was 46 percent. Efficiency may also be measured through ordinarily collected information from community mental health centers. One index might be the ratio of individual to group outpatients, a ratio that was 3.9 in 1970 and 1971. The Biometry Division of NIMH provides a number of indexes like this for community mental health centers. Similar indices could be used for comparisons among other facilities.

Another monitoring form of program evaluation which is tied into reimbursement is accreditation by the Joint Commission on Accreditation of Hospitals. For example, inpatient services at psychiatric institutions for a patient under 21 are authorized for reimbursement if the hospital is accredited and the treatment is active and meets the standards described in the regulations for Title 18 of the Social Security Act as amended.

The impact of this requirement is clear. An article from the *Washington Post* (1973), entitled "State Hospital Loses Rating," ran as follows:

> Physical inadequacies and understaffing uncovered by a January inspection team have lost Spring Grove State Hospital its accreditation, according to the (Maryland) state health department. The Catonsville hospital's head said the action could cost the state as much as $1.75 million in third-party insurance money now being paid by such institutions as Medicare and Blue Cross. Dr. John Hamilton, acting superintendent of the hospital, said such insurors will not pay for care in a non-accredited hospital. He said about one-third of the hospital's 2,000 patients have third-party coverage.

The evaluation involved in accreditation inspection has a lot of motivating power. The impact of funding conditions on quality of care is a topic where little is known and need for knowledge is great. Procedures for evaluative monitoring remain poorly developed, and yet procedures of this sort appear almost inevitable.

Another form of accountability is citizen-group accountability. The National Association of Mental Health has been interested in having their local affiliates conduct what they call "site visitations," visits to the facility to see how responsive it is to community needs. A research grant has been given to Tufts University to develop evaluation procedures that citizen groups might use (MacMurray, et al., 1976).

Another form of program evaluation is the appraisals made by the mass media. This is one of the more effective forms of evaluation. Public exposure of the conditions at a facility or in a program are likely to arouse the public and result in changes.

Let me end with a summary of what I've tried to cover. Figure 2 portrays two bad kinds of program evaluation and suggests two alternative approaches. It seems to me that there is a contest between truth and utilization in program evaluation. Scientific studies are high in truth but low in utilization. Practitioners don't read them. They're not phrased in a way that busy administrators can understand them easily and the practical implications are often not clear. On the other hand, other types of activities that often pass for program evaluation are very high on utilization but frequently low on validity. These are the exposes of programs that may be done for publicity purposes and the public relations efforts by program advocates.

A better compromise between truth and utilization comes from internal evaluation which involves management in planning the program evaluation efforts and feeds back results informally. Such evaluation has more chance for utilization, yet doesn't compromise truth severely.

External evaluation which better combines truth and utilization will come from the new kinds of accountability prompted by

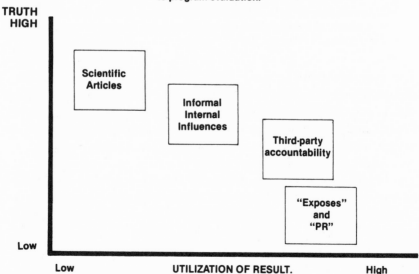

Fig. 2   The trade-off of benefits in four approaches to program evaluation.

changes in the system of financing services. Clearly there will be more utilization. With some research to develop techniques, results should be adequate in validity.

One example of the difficulty of getting program staff to accept the results of external evaluation involves the impact of community mental health centers on state hospital utilization. One of the alleged major initial purposes of the center's program was to channel into community mental health programs people who otherwise would have to go into state mental hospitals.

To test how much community mental health centers have achieved one of the original primary goals of the Community Mental Health Center's Programs, to reduce the state hospital resident rate, Diana Scully and I (1973) did a longitudinal comparison of areas with and without federally funded centers. Sixteen states provided state hospital resident data by county for at least 5 years. For each state, we calculated resident rates each year for counties differing by the year the center opened. The data for Pennsylvania, the largest state in our sample, are shown in Figure 3. There are not large differences between counties with or without centers, nor a consistent change in curves associated with the time when centers opened. Although states differed, overall there seemed no relationship between the opening of centers and change in resident rates. A similar examination for admission rates showed centers may lower state

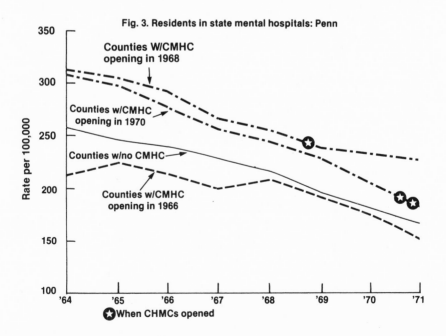

Fig. 3. Residents in state mental hospitals: Penn

hospital admission rates. Thus, centers appear to have more impact on the flow of patients to state hospitals than on the flow of state hospital patients to the community. And the center's program goal of reducing resident rates seems to need additional program emphasis.

When this study was reported to NIMH, there was much disinterest and rejection of the conclusions and their implications. Clearly, these results do not support program rhetoric and suggest that there should be a change in the program and/or its rhetoric. Discussions with NIMH staff revealed a variety of reasons for rejection of the results—some were technical, but more what is termed "political," or special interest serving. It seemed to me that the admission of lack of program achievement was felt by program staff to make the program too vulnerable to attack to be feasible. This "paranoid" interpretation had some support in the actions then being taken by the administration to terminate the centers program. My view, biased by my involvement in the evaluation, was that the negative results should be used as a rationale for program improvement.

Of course, there is another side to this issue as shown by the statistics in Table 1 taken from centers' annual inventories in 1971. These are cross-sectional results. The data reported by each center on the number of people from its catchment area that went to state hospitals were used to calculate the resident rate at state hospitals. This comparison showed that, overall, where you had catchment areas with centers that were reporting the data, the rate was lower than for the United States as a whole. The table shows three different sets of centers; those that were less than a year and a half old, those that were over three years old, and those in between. It's logical to expect that if the centers are having an impact, the difference would be greater for the older centers. These data from the annual inventory fit well what program-supporters want to be able to say at congressional hearings, and have received more attention and citation, even though they make no attempt to measure change, than the longitudinal data from 17 states.

TABLE 1
State Hospital Resident Rates for Center Catchment Areas—1971

Years Center has been open	Rate as Ratio of U.S. Rate
Less than $1\frac{1}{2}$	0.83
$1\frac{1}{2}$ to 3	0.75
over 3	0.71
Total	0.74

It must be said in fairness that the NIMH did try to set up a procedure to make all the information from all of its evaluation studies available to the public routinely. It was felt that the Freedom of Information Act requires government agencies to do this. Making results available routinely partly answers the question of what to do with results. Do you just give them to the program administrator who may shelve them, or do you make special efforts to make results available to the public? Of course, a routine system doesn't fully answer the question, because who in the public gets reports out of the National Technical Information Service? How many people know about the reports? You really have to have a public advocate to dissiminate information like this that would be adverse to the short-run interests of the program—that it should suggest program changes.

This brings me back to where I began with program evaluation. The one thread throughout this discussion, I believe, has been misuse. It seems to me that the system can and should be changed, but it's not the program evaluators' job to change the system; it is the administrators' or the citizens'. I think citizens should insist on getting the information and a high education public policy administrator ought to be concerned with a system that does get information out so that alternative interpretations can be debated.

Since its genesis in seventeenth century England, the scientific method has transformed the West. As a result of a variety of applications to a variety of settings, the scientific method has in fact evolved into a whole range of approaches to experience which bear a family resemblance to one another. Dr. Marcia Guttentag makes an important point in her effort to promote a decision theoretic approach to the evaluation of social programs. The use of Bayesian statistics and subjective probabilities is every bit as scientific as classical hypothesis testing. The critical difference is that the former does not do violence to the organic quality of human service programs. It is the inherent complexity of social settings and dependence upon leadership's ability to size up situations that causes serious problems for the classical approach with its demands for control groups, rigid hypotheses, and overly defined goals. Perhaps the lesson learned in other fields is finally making its way into the applied social sciences, that the situation calls forth the method, so that the method does not transform the situation.

Chapter 19

PROMISING NEW APPROACHES THROUGH THE USE OF BAYESIAN STATISTICS

Marcia Guttentag

A Definition of Evaluation Research

What is evaluation? There's considerable agreement about the definition. Here evaluation is measurement of the desirable and undesirable consequences of an action that has been taken in order to forward some goal that we value. Evaluation research should provide decision makers with sufficient information so that they can: (1) decide whether a program is meeting its objectives, (2) choose between alternative programs or projects and also decide whether to continue existing programs or projects, and (3) receive continuous feedback so that ongoing programs can be improved.

That definition of evaluation research leads to the underlying characteristic of all evaluation, that it eventually leads to a judgement by decision makers about the worth of a program or a set of alternative programs, either actual or conceived. Such final judgments by decision makers are inherently subjective. Their final actions are based on their values and the extent to which data supports their hypotheses about what is actually happening.

The Classical Model

Some evaluation researchers deplore the inherently subjective nature of the evaluation research process and its outcomes. Their approach is to try to purge evaluation research—at least up to the final stage where the decision is made—of what seem to be "unscientific" elements, i.e., the subjectivity of the hypotheses and values of decision makers. This is a basic theme of Ed Suchman's (1967) book on classic evaluation research. He believes that all evaluation research has the form of classical methodology and, as such, must be purged of the inherently subjective values of the decision makers.

> Evaluation research is first and foremost research and as such must adhere as closely as possible to currently accepted standards of classical research methodology. And ultimately the significance of the results must be determined according to the exact same scientific standards used to judge non-evaluative research.

That seems an unobjectionable position. But let us see how it leads to certain consequences about the way in which evaluation research is now practiced.

Are Programs Independent Variables?

Typically what is done in evaluation in the classical experimental (and statistical) approach is to have the decision maker excluded from the research process. An evaluation researcher may initially ask a decision maker what the goals of the program are to help in the formulation of the researcher's hypotheses. Thereafter, he generally is excluded from the research itself. The formulated hypotheses are then translated by the researcher so as to conform as closely as possible to a classical experimental format, null-hypothesis testing, and experimental control groups. The strongest assumption is that social action programs or projects are analogous to independent variables. (If a program is assumed to be an independent variable, it must be the same over time and place, or at least reasonably consistent.) Change in programs, therefore, are prevented wherever possible, so as to make sure that the independent variable remains the same over time.

Pre- and postmeasurement is typical of this approach. Continuous measurement is rare. Often, preposterous assumptions of randomness are made. Classical tests of significance appropriate to answering "is there a difference" questions about infinite populations from small random samples are the statistical methods that are usually used.

Questioning the Classical View of Evaluation

Two groups of serious objections to this evaluation research ap-proach have been made. One body of objections comes from consumers of evaluation, including program administrators/program personnel, and decision makers, local and national. Another group of objections come from the evaluation researchers themselves; both deserve examination.

Most programmers believe that researchers assume action pro-grams should be designed to achieve more specific ends than program administrators had in mind. The researchers tend to narrow outcomes in order to deal with manageable measures, behavioral objectives, for example. The programmers are uneasy with the idea that the success of action programs can be defined by specific and often narrowly defined measures. Frequently, it is only the recipients of programs who are the subject of measurement, rather than the broader, perhaps less defined groups and institutions in which the programmers are interested. Changes in institutions are usually unmeasured. Programmers also question the analogy between a social program and a laboratory experiment. Another objection is that studies often have little to offer to anyone who must make decisions about changes in ongoing programs. Evaluation research-ers too often look at outcomes rather than findings that can be used in continuous change of programs. Judgments about the relative worth of programs are difficult to make with only the information from classical evaluation research. Given such evaluation research embarrassments, it is difficult to make decisions about such broad problems as: Which set of alternative programs should receive more funding? Which type of services should receive greater emphasis?

In practice, of course, these kinds of questions are hopelessly reductive, unless asked in terms of specific contexts. Let me illustrate this with the classic horror story in evaluation: the Head Start evaluations of late 1960s. In this case, the Office of Economic Opportunity (OEO) asked: Does Head Start work or doesn't it work? This is a nonsense question because the only question you *can* ask is: What kinds of programs work on what kinds of populations and in what settings? If data are aggregated and all the regional, program and other differences are eliminated, the outcome is a mishmash. It looks as though there are no results. That's essentially what OEO did, and it ended with nothing. You can say from the outset that for any national social treatment program if you ask some such question as, Does it work nationally? The answer will always be no, simply because of aggregation problems; there is no need to bother evaluating the program.

In certain situations, as in medicine, for example, outcomes are clean-cut. In the case of tuberculosis, there is an independent variable, the tuberculosis bacilli, clearly differentiated from everything else. In the case of Head Start, a government official in OEO sending money to different places in the country provides no indication that comparable programs existed, or that there were *any* programs at all. There's no good analogy between a social action program and an independent variable.

An extreme example occurred in New York City, where a group was asked to evaluate Title I programs in the schools. They went to the schools to find out if anybody knew there were Title I moneys, and to see if there were any Title I programs. They found that, in the majority of the schools, no one knew. The money had simply come in and been used for other purposes. Thus, when an official in the Office of Education said, "Let's evaluate the effects of Title I," he made an incorrect assumption, i.e., that money means programs, and that programs are necessarily comparable.

In summary, programmers' concern is that they are not getting what they need to make continuous decisions about the worth of programs, about remedying mistakes and for long- and short-range planning.

What is the evaluation researcher's point of view when he is armed only with classical methodologies and classical statistics (Neyman-Pierson, Fischerian, null-hypothesis testing)? Evaluation researchers find that the context in which they must operate is different from the classical experimental context. They, therefore, do everything they can to shape the program into one in which they can apply the methods they have learned. They try to abstract those few hypotheses that they consider most researchable from the program's broad, and often multi-faceted goals. The specific hypotheses may have relatively little relevance to the actual program goals. Because they don't begin with their own hypotheses, researchers often try to tease hypotheses out of program administrators. (Program administrators usually have goals, not hypotheses.)

The evaluation researcher often does not have any control over what he's studying; it is not a classical experimental situation. Often he cannot randomize subjects or treatments, and he cannot control the flow of subjects into and out of the program. Frequently, when he tries to, conflicts with the program administrator arise. At a conference at the Brookings Institution, some negative income tax evaluation findings were analyzed and critiqued. The findings were largely uninterpretable because subjects had not been randomized. This is a crucial dilemma. Frequently, even when there are control groups, and people talk in terms of quasi-experimental designs, many of the assumptions that are really required are not met.

In a number of large experimental studies of social programs, whole cities are used as control groups, i.e., Pittsburgh, for example, is matched to a city of comparable size. No matter what variables are matched in the two cities, there are many critical variables that cannot be matched, such as the history of these towns, the industries, etc. One is almost always defeated on grounds of external validity.

Faced with the difficulty of not meeting the assumptions required by the models that he uses, the evaluation researcher cannot count on any help from academics and classical statisticians, for they simply exhort him to clean up the research (make it more random) control his subjects better. Compendia of evaluation research conferences are filled with these exhortations.

Faced with the difference between a real situation and what he's told to do, the evaluation researcher has two choices: He may choose a relatively superficial aspect of the program to study—one which is most vaguely analogous to a single treatment, from which he can obtain some limited behaviorial measures. Or he abandons the pretense of obtaining data that can be fitted into the classical model and turns to a solely descriptive strategy. He becomes a participant-observer and uses anthropological methods or just gives decision makers a vast amount of descriptive material.

Both these strategies lead to frustration for the decision maker. Even when he has a great deal of descriptive material, he doesn't have anything that even indirectly is germane to decision making. A limited study that uses classical methods, does not provide sufficient materials relevant to the broad goals of the program.

An Alternative Evaluation Research Model

As almost everyone else in my generation, and like those in previous generations, I was trained to believe that only one scientific model was acceptable for making inferences and only one statistical system, the classical, could be used. But there are alternative models for making inferences, and there are fortunately alternative statistical systems that make very different assumptions about the nature of the data. One should choose between alternative models with their statistical systems to best fit the nature of the problem. In evaluation research, it is the judgment of the worth of programs which decision makers must make that is crucial. A conceptual model should be used that permits the value and goals of decision makers to be specified and quantified. The statistical system used in evaluation should handle the inherently subjective nature of the hypotheses of decision makers, and it should be data-inclusive. Decision theoretic methods, particularly multiattribute utilities and Bayesian statistics, provide a conceptual framework and statistical methods which fit the natue of the evaluation research problem.

One interested in finding out the extent to which programs do or do not fulfill the multiple values and goals of decision makers should take a multimethod and multivalued approach.

The Sources of Multiple Values in Social Programs

In every social action program, there are many decision makers and many others (e.g., congressional committees, program administrators, recipients of programs, social agencies which deliver the programs) whose values and goals are in some way related to it, as well as concerned outside groups that feel that the program impinges on their interests. Evaluation research methods should characterize and quantify the values and goals of these diverse groups and should provide feedback on the extent to which programs meet their values and goals. Classical methods cannot accomplish these ends; decision theoretic methods can.

Need for Continuous Feedback in Evaluation

Evaluation research requires continuous feedback. It should be possible to change programs daily, weekly, monthly, or at whatever rate the programmers desire. Although it is theoretically possible to use classical null-hypothesis testing to provide continuous feedback by chopping down the pre-/post- null-hypothesis unit into tiny little segments, it is not the way that methodology is used. Most null-hypothesis tests assume that the program is stable over time, and that researchers must wait for a long period before they provide any feedback.

Bayesian statistics permit continuous feedback at any time, because this is built into the methodology; the revision of hypotheses is unconnected with data-gathering operations.

Methods that provide continuous feedback without imposing constraints on programs, i.e., which permit a program to change as much as people want it to change, are critical in evaluation research. So are methods that permit decision makers to revise their values and goals, as well as their probabilities about the state of nature, and to integrate the two. Also, evaluation should be linked to the planning process so as to insure the relevance of evaluation research decisions. Often they are conducted separately. Decision theoretic methods, (multiattribute utilities) combined with Bayesian statistics fulfill the conditions.

Decision Theoretic Methods

Decision theoretic approaches deal with the decision makers' subjective answers to two questions: What is at stake? What are the odds? The answer to the latter requires either direct estimation of probabilities or the kind of information processing for which Bayesian statistics is the optimal mathematical model. The question of what's at stake, i.e., the values or goals, requires the measurement of values or utilities. Utilities, as defined in decision theory, are both the negative and positive properties assessed as the result of a course of action. Each possible course of action has its own set of utilities. One can determine across the whole set of utilities which will provide the maximum outcome for decision makers.

Decision theoretic multiattribute utilities provide the conceptual framework for evaluation, providing the conceptualization and quantification of the values and goals of decision makers. They substitute for what, in classical research, would be considered the goals of the program.

Bayesian statistics are used in the evaluation of what in fact is happening. The data serve as a base in terms of which the hypotheses of decision makers are revised. The conceptual framework is provided by the Multiattribute Utilities System (MAUT), and a way of handling data by the use of Bayesian statistics. The evaluation framework proposed here, links the two.

Edwards' MAUT Methodology

There are nine steps in the Edwards' application of the MAUT system.

1. Identify the organization whose utilities are to be maximized. You must of course specify how utilities from the organization will be obtained. For an organization as large as a whole society, you would need to specify which groups would be included. Probably your focus would be narrowed to a set of groups or organizations.
2. Identify the issue or issues to which the needed utilities are relevant. What is it you want to examine?
3. Identify the entities to be evaluated. An entity is any course of action or program which decision makers must evaluate.
4. Identify the relevant dimensions of value. This requires you to decide which groups you are going to deal with.
5. Rank the value dimensions in order of importance. This ranking is done by the representatives of the decision-making organizations. Different groups may show different ranks. It's uncomfortable to try to rank-order values of different kinds. It is like apples, oranges, and elephants thrown together.
6. Rate the value dimensions in importance while preserving the ratios. Suppose the lowest rank is 10, then judgments up the value hierarchy will have this as a base. A set of weighted values of importance will result.
7. The importance weights are summed, and each is divided by the sum. Normalized importance weights result.
8. The location of each evaluated entity for each dimension is measured. A matrix is created in which weighted values of importance head each column and entities are placed in each row. On a scale of 0 to 100 or 0 to 1000, the decision makers' subjective probabilities about the extent to which each entity maximizes each value will provide a location measure to be put in each cell of the matrix. For example, to what extent do national Head Start programs maximize the likelihood that children will show gains in self-respect and gains in respect for other ethnic groups (the value or goal)? Experts tell us that on a scale of 0 to 100, it's probably 50, which will then be the location measure for that cell. Or, when considering the question whether national Head Start maximizes the potential short-term effects, they may give a location measure of 75 for that cell. One goes across the entire set of values, making prior probability judgments about the extent to which the entity maximizes each value. This is a thoroughly subjective process, a way of providing numbers for what is ordinarily subjective.

9. The next step is the calculation of utilities for each entity using the formula: $U_i = {}_jw_j u_{ij}$ remembering that: ${}_jw_j = 100u_i$ is the aggregate utility for the ith entity. w_j is the normalized importance weight of the jth dimension, and u_{ij} is the rescaled position of the ith entity on the jth dimension. Thus, w_j emerges from step 7, and u_{ij} emerges from step 8. Each entity has a summed utility which represents the weight of a value times the probability that the entity is maximizing that value. An overall utility for each entity results. It tells us, in terms of our current values and what we think various programs are actually doing, which entities are most closely maximizing our values.

From Planning to Evaluation

The basic aim of the evaluation is to change the numbers in each cell of a matrix from absolutely subjective prior probabilities to posterior probabilities based on data. Using Bayesian statistics, one gathers data using these numbers in the cells as prior probabilities. The numbers are then revised, based on what is actually found in the real world.

One is immediately forced into a multiple-method approach because, if probabilities for every one of the values must be revised, measurements that are appropriate to every one of these values must be obtained. If, for example, you are doing an evaluation of Head Start, measurements must be obtained on the extent to which children's self-respect is changed, if that is one of your values. To operationalize that construct requires several methods of measuring how children's self-respect is changed. If there are 15 values, there would be a minimum of 15 operational measures. Sometimes there are as many as 30 or 40 different measures for a social program. The data are then used to provide numbers to replace the completely subjective judgments. In using Bayesian statistics, you are always revising decision makers' prior probabilities with data. His posterior probabilities are based on the data provided.

Note that this is not null-hypothesis testing. Perhaps the decision maker has a null-hypothesis hunch. If he does, then it is tested. Frequently decision makers do not name such hypotheses. It is their hypotheses, whatever they are, for which data is gathered.

$$\frac{P(H_a)}{P(H_b)} \frac{P(D/H_a)}{P(D/H_b)} = \frac{P(H_a/D)}{P(H_b/D)}$$

The first term is prior odds, i.e., the ratio of the probability of hypothesis A to the probability of the hypothesis B before anything is observed. That provides the prior probability. The middle term is the likelihood ratio, i.e., the ratio of the probability of observing D if hypothesis A is true, to the probability of observing D if hypothesis B is true. The likelihood ratio is a measure of the degree of discrimination between hypothesis A and hypothesis B provided by a given datum. The prior odds and the likelihood ratio combine into the posterior odds, i.e., the ratio of the probability of hypothesis A to hypothesis B after the datum D has been observed.

Bayesian statistics provide posterior probabilities based on measures. Thus, the completely subjective prior probabilities were changed into posterior ones based on data. The prior may be wrong. Head Start, for example, may have no effect on any measure of the enhancement of children's self-respect. The posterior probability would then go down to zero. If this is so, when utilities for Head Start are refigured, they will be different. Decisions are revised, given data.

Rules for data gathering and the rules for the revision of hypotheses are separated in the Bayesian system. Hypotheses can be revised on a daily or a weekly or a monthly basis. One can ask, "Given the data I have today, what does this mean?" You can stop gathering data at any time. You may say, "Now that I've gathered this much data, I'm not interested in any more." The system permits continuous data gathering. Of course, values can change as well as probabilities. For example, it may be impossible to gather data about certain values. The probabilities in that cell cannot be changed. The decision maker can say, "I am going to hang on to that value" or "Since I can't obtain measures for it, I'm going to throw it away." The process also permits people to revise their values. Decision makers may say, "Even if I cannot obtain any data for it, it is still my most important value."

If there is a change in values, or importance weights, there are different overall utilities for each program. Using this method, the same data can be fed back to groups with different values. They will come to quite different conclusions. Let us presume that Head Start parents have a low importance weight for enhancing children's self-respect but have a high importance weight for making families more independent. When the data shows that Head Start does not enhance children's self-respect, but does make families feel more important, their values will be served by the program. A group which had different values might not be.

Section V

PROSPECTIVES

Chapter 20

A VALUE NEXUS FOR HUMAN SERVICES

Ru M. Sabre
Theodore Vallance

Our society is in a transitional stage from a growth-oriented society to one in which our social and economic institutions have to adjust to a steady or diminishing supply of energy and raw materials. The stresses and social breakdowns of a bustling expanding economy are being replaced by the stresses and social breakdowns of the adjustments of a myriad of organizations cutting back and reevaluating their goals. Executives are being fired in midcareer, large plants are idling workers for months at a time, managers are making heartbreaking decisions. Among the results of these changes and stresses are child and wife abuse, alcoholism, suicide, nervous collapse, physical illness, drug abuse, broken homes, and an occasional smug attitude on the part of those who through luck have avoided these problems.

Of the many variables that are common among the various forms of social breakdown, we focus on the loss of positive self-regard. Whether this has been caused by ill health, a nervous breakdown, the loss of a job, or being arrested, the net result is a personal devaluation. Further, we hold that this loss of self-regard severely handicaps the individual in efforts to be meaningfully and gainfully employed. These people are cut off from not only the good life, but often from positive and supportive social contacts and interactions. They are alienated.

The value system of any society indicates how rewards and punishments are distributed to people. A utilitarian ethic rewards any activity in accord with the maxim: "the greatest good for the greatest number." Its implications of democratic processes whereby the determination and distribution of goods are made through a process of majority rule are apparent. This ethic and the associated Protestant work ethic evolved in eighteenth and nineteenth century England and was the rationale for the many transformations of English society from a pastoral to an industrial basis. Larger quantities of cheaper goods meant more people would be clothed and fed. Utilitarianism was the ethic of growth capitalism. This ethic reached its logical and fullest expression with the social Darwinism of the late nineteenth century and the early twentieth century. This view of society implies that the human race is essentially two species, one human, the other subhuman. The humans or people are those who can function and be productive in an industrial state. Those who cannot function in an industrial state become identified as subhumans. They are most commonly known as losers, washouts, those who can't cut it, weirdos, beatniks, bums, and so forth. The subhumans were seen as nonproductive excess baggage, and "If you don't work, you don't eat."

From the utilitarian perspective people are sorted out in an either/or fashion. A refinement of this view was the category of the "worthy" poor. These were the individuals who were known to have been unlucky. They "deserve" the charity of others. However, in an urban setting with its relative personal anonymity, if you are poor and out of work or sick or have been arrested, few with power know you and call you worthy and therefore deserving.

At the time that utilitarianism was evolved, a competing social ethic began. This was the social contract view of man's relationship to society. This view, attributed mainly to Rousseau, has it that civilization is the cause of man's ills. People should enter into society under the assumption that there is a mutual obligation among all people to help one another. All people are "written into" society.

Historically utilitarianism and the social contract view of society became entangled in the great ideological dispute between capitalism and socialism. However, history has proven that socialism can imply utilitarian views, and capitalism can imply social contract views of man's relationship to man. One need only study the Soviet Union's treatment of minorities and Sweden's welfare state to see that this is the case. Today, our society has a value structure that is a mixture of utilitarianism and the social contract. We have many features of a welfare state, yet there is a strong sentiment of opposition to the "bleeding hearts" who espouse a social contract view of our obligation to our fellow man. We feel it imperative to declare a social contract view of ethics as the ethics of human services and make clear what this entails in terms of perceivable outcomes.

A social contract view of human services entails a developmental more than a remedial view of human problems, a conviction that the family and community are the primary loci of help, and belief in the value of a partnership between federal, state, and local levels of government with regard to financing and managing human services. What is required is a shift in the perception of the origin and nature of social problems, the locus of change, and the role of government. The key value change is from a treatment view of social problems to a developmental view. The developmental view espouses the establishing of goals for human growth and of the means for making such growth possible, and states that setbacks should be viewed as learning experiences for both the society and the individual. Misfortunes should become a basis for reintegration into society. This means that no one has the right to prevent someone from benefiting from his own mistakes.

To make these values clear, we present a model of society which points to features that make society both the instrument of personal fulfillment for some and an engine of destruction for others. The model is expressed in terms of six propositions each of which will be expanded upon. The basic propositions are:

1. Positive self-regard is a delicate balance of freedom and responsibility.
2. Each person is pursuing his own good.
3. Each place of employment is pursuing its own good.
4. A conflict of individual and organizational objectives results in there being fewer jobs than people.
5. The federal government alone is an inadequate protector of the defenseless.
6. The human services should adopt an advocacy role for their clientele and be active agencies of social change.

Positive Self-Regard Is a Delicate Balance of Freedom and Responsibility

Work simultaneously implies a self-fulfillment and self-denial. A person is free to the degree that his chosen activities allow him to provide for himself both necessities and some tantalizing frills. Underlying these facts are the more fundamental ones that the environment has to be predictable enough to guarantee that activities will be rewarded or punished.

Self-denial and self-fulfillment simultaneously exist in choices that are made. This is best seen in the schematic presented in Figure 4.

There is a curvilinear relationship between order and freedom. Under a condition of zero social order, freedom is nonexistent; there could be no basis for predicting the consequences of choice—and hence no meaning for choosing—in a random universe. At the opposite extreme, complete order precludes deviation from behavior established by the fully ordered system. The gears in a clock can ony turn; they cannot leave. We propose that the same curvilinear relationship exists for the individual person, for he, too, is a structured system.

Why should individual freedom be found greatest in the central portion of the order—disorder range? The individual in a reasonably ordered society "earns his rights" to education, protection, and the other amenities afforded, by demonstrating (or "conforming to") accepted social norms. The various patterns of social interaction are maintained through an exchange of benefits between people.

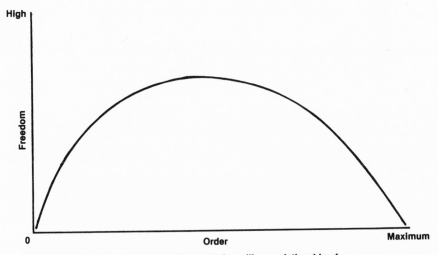

Fig. 4. Suggested curvilinear relationship of
order and freedom.

Each Person Is Pursuing His Own Good

Thus, our society emphasizes individual initiative and self-protection as virtues. The process of maturation is the recognition that this self-guidance is charted with the interests of others in mind. We have the *obligation* to order our own lives, and life and society provide us with guideposts which point in the direction of what is deemed the good life, a life whose activity benefits the individual and society. Career development proceeds on faith at the earlier high school or under-graduate level and is gradually replaced by calculated utility which encompasses the needs of society.

Today, the average person will typically change his career about three times. Successful changes are typically marked by increases in status and income while unsuccessful changes are marked by a decrease in status and income. The trauma of a seriously unsuccess-ful change is hard for a person who has not experienced one to imagine. Built into our social system is an unstable, skilled, semi-skilled, and unskilled labor market. The fate of this average blue collar worker and his family seems to be at the whim of the market and other conditions beyond his control.

In effect, while the individual attempts to order his life and pursue the best for himself and his loved ones, the way society is ordered constrains his ability to choose.

Each Place of Employment Is Pursuing Its Own Good

Any organization has a staff that reflects the needs of that organiza-tion. These needs can change with changes in technology and the market. All "places" of employment are environments where one's decisions are more fully shaped to conform to the needs of others making up the organization. Thus, freedom and responsibility are fused and positive self-regard is fostered in the pursuit of one's own good while contributing to the good of others. But for the "good of the organization," some people are fired or otherwise eliminated from it. A person might be replaced for a variety of reasons, but most times it is not for incompetence.

A Conflict of Individual and Organizational Objectives Results in There Being Fewer Jobs than People

Our economy is so arranged that there will always be a sizeable section of the work force that will be unemployed. Normally this section comes to 3 to 5 percent, though in times of economic recession its size may come to 7 or 8 percent of the work force. The reasons for a pool of unemployed are many and include voluntary resignation, being mobile between jobs, technological replacement of human labor, illness, and constant effort of management to reduce costs of production in a competitive economy. Whatever the figure at any time, for that percent of the population, a fundamental and necessary condition of positive self-regard is removed. A social contract view of social justice, plus various religion-based ethics, asserts that governments are obligated to provide for and protect this population. Further, since our society chooses to motivate individuals on the basis of status and financial enhancement as fundamental values, the loss of status and income provide artifically induced trauma. One is astounded at the contempt expressed for a white collar person who will not readily accept a production line job.

The Federal Government Alone is an Inadequate Protector of the Defenseless

In its period of consolidation since being created under the Eisenhower administration, the U.S. Department of Health, Education and Welfare has spent hundreds of billions of dollars to improve the lot of American citizens. One basic lesson of the last 25 years is that a centrally dictated human service effort is not sufficient to provide for the sick, the mentally ill, the unemployed, the hungry, the malnourished, and the many who do not or cannot succeed, adapt, or develop and who are themselves unhappy and miserable, and who are sources of unhappiness and misery for others. These people represent a very large total of many kinds of social costs.

The various social action programs of the 1960s represented a turning point in the federal government's perception of ameliorating social ills. The general recognition is that the family and the community are properly the locus of most forms of social rehabilitation. Although this is not a return to the Elizabethan poor laws of 1603, which would cause the indigent person to be returned to his place of birth, the current federal philosophy is attempting to strengthen aspects of the local social structure so that it can better cope with the problems of the welfare population, the physically and mentally ill, law breakers, vagrant youth, and elderly poor.

The people who have not experienced any of the variety of social disappointments tend to label those who have with some defect of character and to think of them as in trouble because of bad choices or weakness of will. The social contract view tends to weigh circumstances more heavily and to distinguish a third category somewhere between being saved and being damned, a purgatory where rebirth comes out of disappointment. The social contract perspective takes the scientific view, requiring us to examine social disadvantage more closely and distinguish its various types and causes. The social contract view is realistic, in that it holds that our society has wrongly isolated itself from the harsh realities of life, from the deformed and mentally retarded, the elderly poor, the mentally ill. The family and the community are the place for these.

The value implications of a social contract ethics for human services are simple and profound. The family and community as the locus of help implies that a reaffirmation of the partnership between the federal, state, and local levels be implemented. Local autonomy should be encouraged with a blending of publicly and privately financed services, including especially the volunteer organization. Indeed, this seems to be the trend with the new health legislation dictating a greater decision making responsibility on the part of state and within-state regions. The block grant with general revenue sharing could provide greater flexibility in human service programs. The developmental view of human problems calls for reevaluation of growth-economy values based on large profits and status incentives. Competition and compassion need not be mutually exclusive.

The Human Services Should Adopt an Advocacy Role for their Clientele and be Active Agencies of Social Change

We have asserted a curvilinear relationship of freedom and order, that a measure of individual freedom is a measure of quality of life, and have claimed that freedom can be maximized by maintaining a moderate degree of order. What does this imply for selecting attributes and objectives of mental health and other human service systems? We believe that holding this view of freedom and its relation to social order, including the ensured opportunity to increase through participation in the social order, implies two major propositions:

1. The human services should be designed primarily to optimize chances for individual development rather than to provide remedial services for people.

2. Considering the functions of a society as a whole, the human services should be basic instruments of social change, rather than the means whereby particular social pathologies are attended to.

In other words, we opt for a developmental view of the individual and his problems and of society rather than one that emphasizes ills, pathologies, and their treatments as the guide for emphasis in the further development and evaluation of human services.

A developmental approach does not exclude programs designed to "prevent" particular "illnesses," as a general medical approach might be designed to prevent smallpox through inoculation, or dysentery through better sewage and water filtration systems. A developmental approach is itself more inclusive and more elusive at its present stage of evolution. It seeks to identify and create conditions including organizational and associational forms that will foster more wholesome development, more individual independence and competency through social living, the establishing of clearer goals and more realistic aspirations, and more relevant work habits. In this form of "prevention," the emphasis is on identifying and intervening in conditions that are associated with suboptimal development of human behavioral potential, e.g., malnutrition, poverty, hostile family members, parents who don't know how to raise happy and self-respecting children, heritable or otherwise biologically based inabilities to cope, severely constraining organizational forms, and other conditions leading to alienation and undue stress and anxiety.

Research supporting a developmental form of intervention proceeds on the assumption that conditions of life can be discovered and arranged so as to foster the development of personal skills, attitudes, and abilities, such that later conditions of life will not bring about serious or prolonged and costly dysfunction. Developmental intervention may thus reduce needs for specialized care, such as rehabilitation, correction, treatment, incarceration, or other processes associated with our institutional ways of coping with deviations from social norms that offend and disgust people who want the norms maintained.

Clearly this assertion of the advantages of a developmental approach to designing human services could be bolstered by further argument that would draw upon existing literature on the social and economic costs of existing social problems (e.g., drug abuse, child neglect, alcoholism) and the potential benefits to be gained from preventing them. It certainly should be tested by careful research and demonstrative experiments that would be based on the *most careful statement* of premises as to what the "good life" is for the people to be affected and of measurable indicators of its presence.

Of the several features of the Community Mental Health Centers, as developed on the basis of the Community Mental Health Act of 1963, the most forward looking from the perspective of this book, was the requirement for consultation and education—getting the rest of the community involved with the concept, the problems, and the processes for promoting mental health. It has been this feature of the Community Mental Health program that has given impetus to the study and clarification of the role which the rest of the community—police, schools, social work agencies, homes for the aged, volunteer agencies like Kiwanis and Rotary and many others—could and should have in the promotion of new opportunities for coping with deviant behavior and for reducing the chances of its serious occurrences through promoting the development of more healthy and constructive conditions of community life.

Looking at mental health particularly, we see it as a fundamental indicator of general societal well-being. It is the common experience of mental health centers to trace down such things as child and wife abuse, psychotic episodes, suicides, and other "pathologies" not simply to individual problems in intrapsychic development, but to such things as poor housing, job loss, debt, failure—in short to political, economic, and environmental causes. People in mental health facilities are the worst possible outcomes of societal arrangements.

Even if one accepts as reasonable a developmental view of the human services as we have detailed it, questions can still be asked: But should this really become their job? *Should* the helping services become advocates of the extensive social reforms that would be needed to produce a society that is generally "prodevelopmental" and "anti-Shiva" as the one we would like to see? And given the tax-supported nature of most of them, *can* they become effective agencies of social reform, overcoming political antagonisms that such efforts at reform are certain to provoke? And conversely, why not leave the needed sociopolitical reform to the "normal political process" and the ballot box?

These are reasonable and challenging questions indeed and we will not try to answer them here in detail. However, our position in general is, yes, the human services should continue to be agents of social change and political reform. Why? Because (1) they are mostly peopled by workers of humanitarian interest; (2) they contain the most complete knowledge of the problems of development and hence of the potential benefits in their solutions; (3) they exist as organized constituencies for themselves and for thousands of people who could join in support of their efforts; (4) they contain large numbers of people skilled in as well as dedicated to community action that can supply the political force; and (5) by continuing to do well the helping services they are chartered to do, and adding (after suitable further education and staff development) various developmental approaches to these operations and objectives, they can over time demonstrate what can be done through agency and political action to enhance human potential in modern life.

References

Bennett, C., Anderson, L., Cooper, S., Hassol, L., Klein, D., & Rosenblum, G. (Eds.) *Community psychology*. Boston: Boston University Press, 1966.

Broder, D. S. Presidential power: An interview with Casper W. Weinberger. *Washington Post*, February 18, 1973.

Brown B. S. Address before the joint convention of the Tennessee legislature. Nashville, Tennessee, March, 1973.

Buchanan, G. N., & Wholey, J. S. Federal level evaluation. *Evaluation*, 1972, **1**, 17–22.

Glaser, E. M., & Taylor, S. H. Factors influencing the success of applied research. *American Psychologist*, 1973, **28**, 140–146.

Harvey, E. C. *Sources of funds of community mental health centers*. Report to National Institute of Mental Health from Stanford Research Institute on Contract HSM-42-69-101, Accession No. PB-211-333. Springfield, Va.: National Technical Information Service, 1970.

Health Services and Mental Health Adminstration. *Toward a systematic analysis of health care in the United States*. DHEW Publication No. (HSM) 73-25. Supt. of Documents: Washington, D.C.: U.S. Government Printing Office, 1972.

Kelly, J. G., Boone, D., Newbrough, J. R., & Rooney, H. L. Alternate mental health services for an elementary class nonachieving children. Presented at the American Public Health Association Meetings, Detroit, Michigan, November 16, 1961.

Kelly, J. G., DiMento, J., & Gottlieg, B. S. The community as teacher. In D. M. Flournoy (Ed.), *The new teachers*. San Francisco: Josey-Bass, 1972, Chap. 16, pp. 170–179.

Kelly, J. G., Snowden, L. S., & Monoz, R. F. Social and community interventions. In *Annual review of psychology*, Vol. 28. Palo Alto, Ca.: Annual Reviews, 1976.

Kelman, H. *A time to speak*: *On human values and social research*. San Francisco: Josey-Bass, 1968.

Klein, D. Community dynamics & mental health. New York: John Wiley, 1968.

Lippitt, R. *The dynamics of planned change*. New York: Harcourt Brace Jovanovich, 1958.

MacMurray, V. D., Cunningham, P. H., Cater, P. B., Swenson, N., & Bellin, S. S. *Citizen evaluation of mental health services*: *A handbook for accountability*. New York: Behavioral Publications, 1976.

Macro Systems, Inc. *Trends in sources of funds for community mental health centers.* Report Health Services and Mental Health Administration on Contract HSM-100-72-369, Accession No. PB-240-461. Springfield, Va.: National Technical Information Service, 1973.

Mercer, J. *Labelling the mentally retarded.* Berkeley, Univ. of California Press, 1973.

Mills, R. & Kelly J. Cultural and social adaptations to change: A case example and critique. In S. Golann & C. Eisdorfer (Eds.). *Handbook of community psychology.* New York Appleton, Croft, 1972.

NIMH. *Planning for creative change in mental health services: A distillation of principles on research utilization.* Vols. I and II. *Bibliography with annotations.* DHEW Publications Nos. (HSM) 71-9060 and 71-9061. Washington, D.C.: U.S. Government Printing Office, 1972.

NIMH. *Planning for creative change in mental health services: A manual on research utilization.* DHEW Publication No. (HSM) 71-9059. Washington, D.C.: U.S. Government Printing Office, 1972.

Reiff, R. Mental health manpower and institutional change. In E. Cowen, E. Gardner, & M. Zax (Eds.). *Emergent approaches to mental health problems.* New York: Appleton, 1967.

Reiff, R. Social intervention and the problems of psychological analysis. *American Psychologist,* 1968, **23**, 524–531.

Rosenhan, D. On being sane in insane places. *Science,* 1973, **179**, 250–258.

Ryan, W. *Blaming the victim.* New York: Random House, 1971.

Sarason, S. *The creation of settings in future societies.* San Francisco: Josey-Bass, 1973.

Scully, D., & Windle, C. *An empirical study of the impact of federally funded community mental health centers on state mental hospital utilization.* Report to NIMH on Contract HSM 42-73-70, Accession No. PB-259-365. Springfield, Va.: National Technical Information Service, 1973.

Simon, G. Right to Treatment? *APA Monitor,* 1971.

Suchman, E. *Evaluation research.* New York: Russell Sage, 1967.

Taube, C. A., & Redick, R. W. Recent trends in the utilization of mental health facilities. In J. Zusman & E. F. Bertsch (Eds.). *The future role of the state hospital.* Lexington, Mass.: Lexington Books, 1975, pp. 524–582.

Washington Post, April 1, 1973. Unsigned.

Wilson, J. State hospital loses rating. *Washington Post,* February 18, 1973.

Windle, C., & Bates, P. Evaluating program evaluation: A suggested approach. In P. O. Davidson, F. W. Clark, & L. A. Hamerlynck (Eds.). *Evaluation of behavioral programs: in community, residential and school settings.* Champaign, Ill.: Research Press, 1974, pp. 395–435.

Windle, C., Bass., R., & Taube, C. PR Aside—Initial results from NIMH's service program evaluation studies. *American Journal of Community Psychology,* 1974, **2**, 311–327.

World Health Organization. *Constitution.* Geneva, 1946.

INDEX